D1587029

Practical Guide to VIVA and OSCE in Ophthalmology Examinations

Practical Guide to VIVA and OSCE in Ophthalmology Examinations

Wei Yan NG

MBBS, MMED (Ophthal)
Singapore National Eye Centre, Singapore

Li Lian FOO

MD, MMED (Ophthal), FRCOphth
Singapore National Eye Centre, Singapore

Tien Yin WONG

MBBS, MMED (Ophthal), MPH, PHD,
FECSE, FRANZCO, FAMS
Singapore National Eye Centre, Singapore

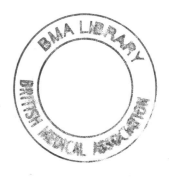

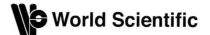

World Scientific

NEW JERSEY · LONDON · SINGAPORE · BEIJING · SHANGHAI · HONG KONG · TAIPEI · CHENNAI · TOKYO

Published by

World Scientific Publishing Co. Pte. Ltd.

5 Toh Tuck Link, Singapore 596224

USA office: 27 Warren Street, Suite 401-402, Hackensack, NJ 07601

UK office: 57 Shelton Street, Covent Garden, London WC2H 9HE

Library of Congress Cataloging-in-Publication Data

Names: Ng, Wei Yan, author. | Foo, Li Lian, author. | Wong, Tien Yin, author. |
    Complemented by (expression): Wong, Tien Yin. Ophthalmology examinations review. 3rd ed.
Title: Practical guide to viva and OSCE in ophthalmology examinations /
    Wei Yan Ng, Li Lian Foo, Tien Yin Wong.
Description: New Jersey : World Scientific, 2018. | Complemented by
    The ophthalmology examinations review / Tien Yin Wong, Wesley Guang Wei Chong,
    Zhu Li Yap, Saadia Farooqui. 3rd edition. 2018. | Includes index.
Identifiers: LCCN 2017044677| ISBN 9789813221512 (hardcover : alk. paper) |
    ISBN 9813221518 (hardcover : alk. paper) | ISBN 9789813221550 (pbk. : alk. paper) |
    ISBN 9813221550 (pbk. : alk. paper)
Subjects: | MESH: Eye Diseases | Ophthalmologic Surgical Procedures | Examination Questions
Classification: LCC RE50 | NLM WW 18.2 | DDC 617.7--dc23
LC record available at https://lccn.loc.gov/2017044677

British Library Cataloguing-in-Publication Data
A catalogue record for this book is available from the British Library.

For any available supplementary material, please visit
http://www.worldscientific.com/worldscibooks/10.1142/10547#t=suppl

Printed in Singapore

CONTENTS

ABOUT THE AUTHORS

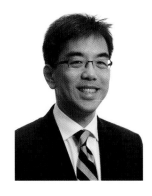

Wong Tien Yin is currently Provost's Chair Professor of Ophthalmology and Medical Director at the Singapore National Eye Center, Duke-NUS Medical School, National University of Singapore. Prof. Wong has served previously as the Singapore Eye Research Institute (SERI) Executive Director (2009–2013), and is currently the Chairman of SERI's Board. Prior to these roles, Prof. Wong was Head of the Department of Ophthalmology, National University of Singapore, and Chair of Department of Ophthalmology, Royal Victorian Eye and Ear Hospital, the University of Melbourne, Australia. Prof. Wong has published >1000 peer-reviewed papers, given >300 invited named, plenary, and symposium lectures globally, and is a two times recipient of the Singapore Translational Researcher Award (2008 and 2014), the highest award for the most senior clinician-scientists in Singapore. Prof. Wong serves on Editorial Boards of *Investigative Ophthalmology and Visual Sciences, JAMA-Ophthalmology, Diabetes Care, Ophthalmologica*, and the *Journal of Hypertension*. He was previously the Executive Editor of the *American Journal of Ophthalmology*. He is a Board member of the National Medical Research Council, a Council member of the Asia Pacific Academy of Ophthalmology and President of the College of Ophthalmologists in Singapore. For his service, Prof. Wong has been recognized nationally and internationally with numerous awards, such as the National Clinician Scientist Award and the President's Science Award, two of the highest awards in Singapore. He is a recipient of the 2013 Eisenhower Fellowship from the USA.

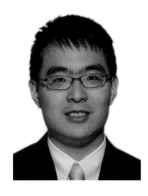

Ng Wei Yan has attained Primary MMED Ophthalmology in 2012, Part 1 FRCOphth in 2013, The Royal College of Ophthalmologists Refraction Certificate in 2014, and Final MMED Ophthalmology in 2016.

Since July 2017, he has been appointed as the Chief Registrar, Singapore National Eye Centre. Other experiences he has include Deputy Lead Resident, Singapore National Eye Centre from February to June 2016, and Lead Resident, Singapore National Eye Centre from July to December 2016.

Dr. Ng has been awarded the NUS Dean's List in 2005, NUS Dean's Dinner in 2005 — 2009, Inspiring Resident Educator Award 2017, and the RISE Award — Quality Improvement Project Award 2017.

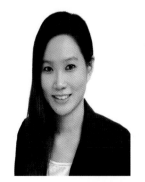

Foo Li Lian *(MD, FRCOphth, MMed (Ophth), BEng (1st class honors))*, graduated from National University of Singapore in 2008 with Bachelor in Engineering (Chemical) — BEng (1st Class Honors). In 2012, she was awarded Doctor of Medicine — MD, by Duke-NUS Graduate Medical School. Her ophthalmology specialization, Fellow Royal College of Ophthalmologist (FRCOphth), and Master of Medicine in Ophthalmology (MMed (Ophth)) were achieved in 2016 and 2017, respectively.

She was awarded NUS Awards for Study Abroad (Exchange Awards) in 2006, Dean's List in 2006, Young Investigator Award (Clinical) in Singapore General Hospital 19th Annual Scientific Meeting in 2011, and the Singapore Society of Ophthalmologists Award for Best Oral Presentation, Runner-Up in 2013.

Dr. Foo has also presented in several conferences, including Paper Presentation at National Ophthalmology Residents' Research Day in 2013, SGH Annual Scientific Meeting, and ARVO Annual Meeting in 2011.

Dr. Foo is currently a senior resident at Singapore National Eye Centre.

LIST OF CONTRIBUTORS

We would like to express our heartfelt gratitude to the following prominent leaders and mentors in Ophthalmology for making this book possible by dedicating their valuable time and resources. Their contributions are sincerely appreciated and gratefully acknowledged.

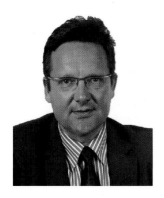

Prof. Dan Milea
MD, PhD

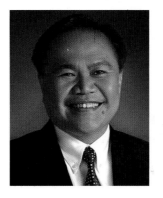

Assoc. Prof. Ian Yeo
MMed(Ophth), FRCS(Ed), FRCSG,
FAMS

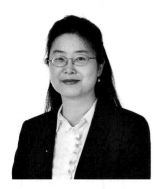

Assoc. Prof. Nga Min En
MBBS, FRCPath, FRCPA, FIAC

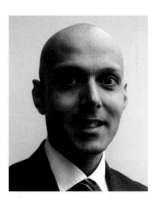

Assoc. Prof. Shamira Perera
MBBS(Hons), BSc(Hons), FRCOphth

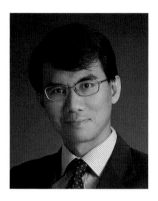

Adj. Assoc. Prof. Quah Boon Long
MMed(Ophth), FRCS(Ed) FAMS

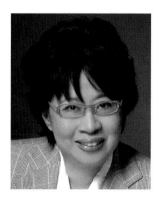

Adj. Assoc. Prof. Seah Lay Leng
MBBS, FRCS(Ed), FRCOphth, FAMS

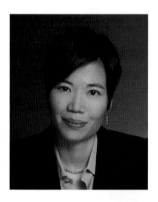

Adj. Assoc. Prof. Sharon Tow
MBBS(Sydney), FRCS(Ed), FAMS

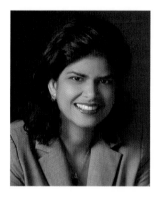

Dr. Anshu Arundhati
MMed(Ophth), FRCS(Ed)

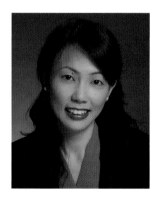

Dr. Loo Jing Liang
MMed(Ophth), FRCS(Ed), FAMS

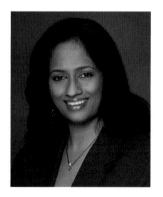

Dr. Ranjana Mathur
MMed(Ophth), FRCS(Ed)

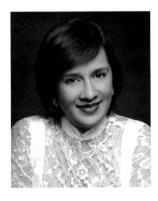

Dr. Sonal Farzavandi
FRCS(Ed)

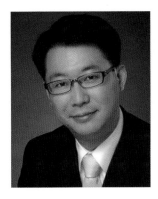

Dr. Sunny Shen
MMed(Ophth), FRCS(Ed), FAMS

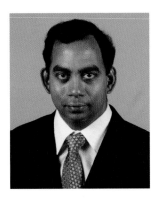

Dr. Thomas Paulraj Thamboo
MBChB, FRCPath, FRCPA

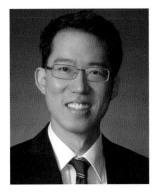

Dr. Laurence Lim
MBBS, FRCS(Ed), FAMS

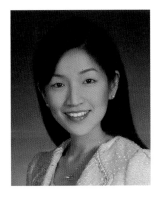

Dr. Livia Teo
MMed(Ophth), FRCS(Ed), FAMS

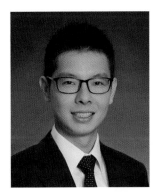

Dr. Andrew Tsai Shih Hsiang
MBBS, MMed(Ophth), FRCOphth,
FAMS

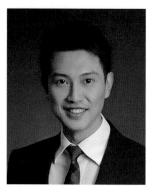

Dr. Daniel Ting
MBBS(1st Hons), BSciMed,
MMed(Ophth) PhD(UWA)

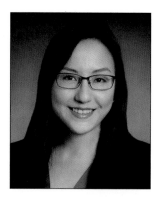

Dr. Yong Kai Ling
MMed(Ophth), FAMS

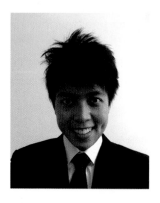

Dr. Val Phua Jun Rong
MBBS, MMed(Ophth)

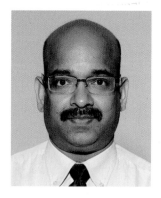

Mr. Kasi Sandhanam
(Senior Ophthalmic Imaging Specialist)

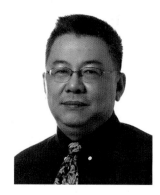

Mr. Joseph Ho Eng Siang
(Principal Ophthalmic Imaging Specialist)

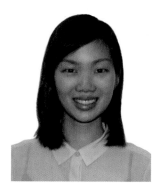

Ms. Ng Lei Yee, Catherine
BHSc and MOrth

CHAPTER 1

CATARACTS

Q **Question 1.1 Viva Stem: How will you Perform Cataract Surgery?**

The most **common cataract surgery** performed in my center is phacoemulsification. I will perform it under informed consent in the operating theater under peribular anesthesia in sterile conditions. Clean and drape and retract the lids with a **Liberman speculum**. Create an **anterior chamber paracentesis and the clear corneal incision 90 degrees apart, continuous curvilinear capsulorrhexis, hydrodissection**, disassembly of the nucleus using **stop and chop technique, irrigation** and **aspiration** of soft lens material. Insert intraocular lens into a viscoelastic inflated bag, remove the viscoelastic, and hydrate the wound with subsequent cefazolin gentamicin dexamethasone spray.

Q **Question 1.2 How would you Define Surge, How do you Reduce Surge, and What are the Phaco Settings that you Use?**

Surge is a result of loss of occlusion under high pressure giving rise to a **rapid rate of fluid exit** from the anterior chamber resulting in a **rise in the posterior capsule**.

It can be controlled **by reducing the compliance of the tubing as well as allowing for venting**. For sculpting, I would use a power of **30 mW** and **30 mmHg** vacuum at a bottle height of **100 cm**. For fragmentation and removal of the nucleus, I will use a power of **20–30 mW** with **300 mmHg** vacuum at a bottle height of **120 cm**. For the last fragment, I will use a power of **15–20 mW** with **180 mmHg** vaccum at a bottle height of **120 cm**. For irrigation and aspiration of soft lens material, I will use **550 mmHg** vacuum at a bottle height **100 cm**.

Q **Question 2 Viva Stem: What are the Considerations in Performing Cataract Surgery in a Patient with APAC Two Days Ago?**

Considerations can be divided into **preoperative, perioperative, intraoperative** and **postoperative.** Preoperatively, I will **control the intraocular pressure** medically in the absence of contraindications, check the **endothelial cell counts** and perform an **ultrasound biomicroscopy** to assess the degree of zonular laxity, **standby anterior vitrectomy,** and obtain **anterior chamber intraocular lens biometry**. If required, I will perform a laser peripheral iridotomy during the acute attack. Perioperatively, I will start the patient on **intravenous mannitol (0.5–2 g/kg)** if the pressure remains high. I will perform the surgery under **peribulbar anesthesia, scrap the epithelium if the view is poor,** create a **longer more anteriorly placed corneal tunnel,** using **soft shell technique** with dispersive viscoelastic to protect the endothelium and cohesive viscoelastic to maintain anterior chamber depth, **refill frequently** but avoiding overfill, performing an *in situ* **chop with a sharp second instrument** to reduce zonular stress, ensuring **complete removal of viscoelastic** at the end of surgery. Postoperatively, I will monitor the intraocular pressure and start the patient on topical antibiotics and steroids.

Q **Question 3.1 Viva Stem: What are the Complications of Cataract Surgery?**

Complications of cataract surgery can be divided into **intraoperative, early and late postoperative** complications. Intraoperative complications include **Descemet membrane detachment, corneal wound burn, iris trauma, capsulorrhexis runout, posterior capsular rupture, dropped nucleus** or **zonulysis,** and **suprachoroidal** or **retrobulbar hemorrhage**. Early postoperative complications include **hypotony from wound leak, hypertony from inadequate viscoelastic removal, corneal edema, infective endophthalmitis, retained lens fragment,** and **toxic anterior segment syndrome.** Late postoperative complications include **retained lens fragment, corneal decompensation, raised intraocular pressure from steroid response, corneal epitheliopathy from antibiotic toxicity, persistent inflammation, posterior capsular opacification, capsular block syndrome, decentered** or **subluxed intraocular lens, refractive surprise, capsular phimosis, cystoid macular edema, retinal tears or detachment,** and **chronic endophthalmitis.**

Q **Question 3.2 Intraoperatively, if you note Shallowing of the Anterior Chamber, what are your Differentials? If there is Sudden Deepening, what are your Differentials?**

When shallowing of the anterior chamber occurs, possible causes include **suprachoroidal hemorrhage, unstable anterior chamber secondary to leaking wound, machine malfunction/irrigation failure** or **aqueous misdirection**. Sudden deepening can result from **lens iris diaphragm retropulsion syndrome, unstable anterior chamber, posterior capsular rupture** or **hydrorupture, zonulysis with lens tilt,** and **increased infusion bottle height.**

Question 4.1 Viva Stem: Describe the Photo Shown in Figure 1.1.

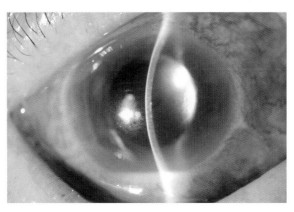

Figure 1.1 This patient has postoperative exogenous endophthalmitis with features of conjunctival injection, hazy cornea, and hypopyon.

This is an anterior segment photograph of the patient's left eye with a slit beam showing a **diffusely injected eye** with **hazy edematous cornea** but **no obvious infiltrates**. There is presence of **hypopyon inferiorly** and the patient is **pseudophakic**. The anterior chamber is **deep** and there are **no obvious lens fragments** present. The pupil is regular with **no obvious vitreous in the anterior chamber** seen. Lid margins appear otherwise normal. This patient likely has a postoperative exogenous endophthalmitis. Other differentials include **retained lens fragment** and **reactivation of underlying uveitis.** (TASS is unlikely in this case as there is no limbal-to-limbal corneal edema.) I will check the **visual acuity** and **light projection** and relative afferent papillary defect, assess for nasolacrimal duct obstruction (as a risk factor for infection) and intraocular pressures, **check the wound for slow leak** (less likely if pressure is high and anterior chamber is deep) and vitreous incarceration, look for posterior capsular rupture under the slit lamp and vitreous in the anterior chamber, and examine the fundus for **vitritis** and **retinal detachment.** If there is no view, I will **perform a B scan** and finally examine the fellow eye for risk factors for operative complications. I will examine the patient's history for the date of surgery, duration and progression of symptoms, compliance to medication and any injury, whether the surgery was complicated and prolonged, and any immunocompromised state.

Question 4.2 A Patient had Cataract Surgery Four Days Ago and now has Vision with only Light Perception. How would you Manage the Patient?

The patient likely has **postoperative exogenous endophthalmitis** until proven otherwise. This is an **ocular emergency**. Management is dependent on **presenting visual**

acuity and presence of **retinal complications** such as detachment. In such a patient with presenting vision of light perception, based on the **Endophthalmitis Vitrectomy Study,** I will refer the patient **urgently** to the vitreoretinal surgeon and organize an **urgent vitrectomy**. If the surgery timing is too far away, I will perform **immediate vitreous tap and jab** in the meantime, sending for gram stain and cultures and injecting intravitreal vancomycin 1 mg in 0.1 mL and ceftazidime 2.25 mg in 0.1 mL in the absence of contraindications, start patient on systemic antibiotics, and admit the patient for monitoring of the progress.

Q **Question 4.3 What are the Risk Factors for Postoperative Endophthalmitis?**

The risks of postoperative endophthalmitis can be split into **patient factors, ocular factors**, and **operative factors.** Patient factors include patients who are immunocompromised such as diabetics, patients who have retroviral infections, patients on immunosuppressive medications, and patients who are non-compliant to eye drops and follow-up visits. Ocular factors include lagophthalmos, exposure, distichiatic lashes, meibomitis, and nasolacrimal duct obstruction. Operative factors include prolonged surgery, wound leak, posterior capsular rupture, dropped nucleus, vitreous adhesion to the wound, or use of silicone lenses.

Q **Question 4.4 What are the Causes of Chronic Endophthalmitis?**

Causes include **propionibacterium acnes, fungal** with an indolent course and **staph epidermidis**.

Q **Question 5 Viva Stem: During Routine Phaco Surgery, you noticed the Anterior Chamber Rapidly Shallowing and Dimming of the Red Reflex. What is your Differential and Management of this Condition?**

The patient is likely to have **suprachoroidal hemorrhage**. This is an **ocular emergency**. Other differentials will include aqueous misdirection and an unstable anterior chamber. **I will stop the surgery and assess immediately, feeling for increased digital pressure and looking for signs of iris and vitreous prolapse.** I will inform the anaesthetist to **start intravenous mannitol 1 g per kg over 20 minutes** in the absence of contraindications and suture the **wound tight with 10/0 nylon**. I will then examine the patient using **indirect ophthalmoscope with a 20 dioptre lens to confirm my diagnosis**. I will start the patient on **maximum topical and systemic glaucoma medications with topical steroids** and cycloplegics. I will refer the patient urgently to the **vitreoretinal surgeon and monitor the patient with daily B scan.**

Risk Factors for Suprachoroidal Hemorrhage

Patient Factors	Ocular Factors	Intraoperative Factors
Elderly	Myopia	Prolonged surgery
Hypertension	Aphakia	Sudden decompression e.g. glaucoma
Cardiovascular disease	Pre-existing glaucoma	Large wounds e.g. ECCE
COPD	Nanophthalmos	PCR
Obesity		Intraoperative tachycardia

Q Question 6 Viva Stem: How will you Perform an Intracapsular Cataract Extraction?

I will perform an intracapsular cataract extraction under informed consent in the operating theater under sterile conditions with peribulbar anesthesia. After cleaning and draping, I will place a **superior bridle suture with 4/0 silk**, perform a **large conjunctival peritomy from** 3 to 9 o' clock (larger than ECCE 10-2) and create **a two-plane limbal incision** from 3 to 9 o'clock. I will first attempt to **manually express the nucleus,** failing which I will attempt to remove using **forceps** and **vectis**. If this also fails, I will then tilt the lens, **dry the area** with a Weck sponge and apply **cryo** to the proximal lens to create adhesions before manually removing the lens (if not, the whole anterior chamber will freeze). I will then perform **anterior vitrectomy** and **create a superior surgical iridectomy**. I can either **insert an anterior chamber intraocular lens** or **leave the patient aphakic for future secondary fixated intraocular lens implant.** I will then close the wound with 10/0 nylon and inject subconjunctival cefazolin, gentamicin, and dexamethasone.

Q Question 7.1 Viva Stem: You are Examining a Patient with Blurring of Vision, Currently one month after a Right Cataract Operation. What are the Causes of Blurring of Vision after a Cataract Operation?

Causes of blurring of vision after a cataract operation can be divided into causes attributable to cataract surgery and other causes. I will first exclude sight-threatening complications such as **endophthalmitis, retinal detachment, bullous keratopathy**, and **steroid-induced glaucoma**. Other causes related to the surgery include topical antibiotic toxicity, prolonged inflammation, reactivation of herpatic uveitis, decentered or subluxed intraocular lens, capsular block syndrome, refractive surprise, posterior capsular opacification and cystoid macula edema (list causes in an anterior to posterior fashion or vice versa).

> **Q** **Question 7.2A Scenario 1: In a Patient with Postop Refraction of -3D in the Right Eye, now noted to have Corneal Thickness of 400 microns, what are the Causes of Inaccuracy of IOL Power Management?**

The patient is likely to have undergone refractive surgery in the right eye. I will examine the left eye for refractive surgery scars and assess the keratometry and refractive error. Refractive surgery results in inaccurate biometry by several methods. Firstly, there is **radius error** as in postrefractive surgery the corneal curvature is altered and the biometry such as the IOLMaster assumes a different radius for calculation (assume a smaller radius). There is also **keratometer error** (overestimated) as most instruments measure only the anterior corneal curvature and assume overall power based on a fixed refractive index of 1.3375 and Gullstrand ratio for peripheral and central cornea (keratometry — overall cornea power). There is also **formula error** which assumes an incorrect lens position based on an incorrect keratometry.

- Radius (too small) → keratometry (too big) → ELP error

Note: IOL formula that can be used for eyes with previous refractive surgeries: haggis-L, Barrett, ASCRS website.

(Approach to refractive surprise: Wrong patient, wrong eye, wrong IOL, wrong biometry.)

> **Q** **Question 7.2B Scenario 2: Postoperatively One Month after Phaco, OCT Showing the following VA 6/15, Management.**

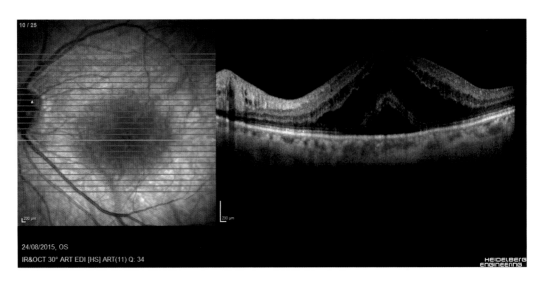

Figure 1.2 Optical coherence tomography of the macula demonstrating the presence of cystoid macula edema centered at the fovea — Irvine–Gass syndrome.

The optical coherence tomography shows large intraretinal cystic thickening involving and centered at the fovea with subretinal fluid. The ellipsoid lines are intact and there is absence of vitreomacular traction. This is possibly **Irvine–Gass macular edema** but I will need to exclude other causes. I will examine the patient's history for any **prolonged cataract operation, compliance to postoperative medications, any complications intraoperatively, vascular risk factors, use of prostaglandin analogues, glaucoma eye drops,** and **retinal dystrophies.** I will check for relative afferent pupillary defect, anterior chamber activity, and retained lens fragment, and for evidence of vitreous loss or posterior capsular rupture, examining the fundus for diabetic retinopathy and central retinal vein occlusion, vasculitis, bony spicules associated with retinitis pigmentosa. I will also examine the contralateral eye. In this patient, in the absence of vitreo-macular traction, management is medical. I will start the patient on **topical steroids and non-steroidal anti-inflammatory drugs,** failing which I will prescribe **oral acetazolamide.** If the cystoid macular edema persists, I will inject either periocular steroids or intravitreal anti-vascular endothelial growth factors. (If there is VMT with vitreous to the wound, consider Yag vitreolysis at the pupil edge or TPPV.)

> Causes of cystoid macular edema (CME)
>
> - most common: Irvine–Gass
> - inflammatory/infective
> - vasculopathy: retinal vein, occlusion, diabetes, hypertension
> - drug: prostaglandin
> - retinal dystrophies: retinitis pigmentosa
> - tractional: epiretinal membrane

Q **Question 7.3 How do you Differentiate Cystoid Macular Edema from DM CSME?**

Differentiating Irvine–Gasse syndrome from clinically significant macular edema can be difficult. I will perform a fluorescein angiogram. In Irvine–Gasse, there will be **a petaloid leakage centered at the fovea with disc staining as compared to diabetic edema which has more diffuse and irregular leakage from the microaneurysms, usually not centered at the fovea** and has disc leakage instead of staining.

Q **Question 8.1 Viva Stem: Intraoperatively during Hydrodissection, you noted Sudden Narrowing of the Pupillary Aperture. What is your Impression and Management of this Condition?**

There is the likely presence of **hydrorupture.** Principles of management would be to **prevent drop nucleus** and **ensure safe delivery of the lens and implantation of an appropriate intraocular lens.** I would call for help and inform the **vitreoretinal surgeon.**

I will then **support the lens via a pars plana approach with injection of viscoelastic,** perform **relaxing incisions on the capsulorrhexis** (using cystotome), following which I will convert to an **extracapsular cataract extraction by extending the wound** (either cornea or sclera) and **delivering the lens with a paediatric Vectis forceps.** I will perform a thorough **anterior vitrectomy** and **removal of cortical material using manual aspiration, implantation of a three-piece intraocular lens into the sulcus** and **miose the pupil with carbechol,** then **suture the wound with 10/o nylon ensuring watertight closure.** I will then perform a final check of the wound to ensure no vitreous adhesion. I will start the patient on topical antibiotics and steroids in the absence of contraindication **with oral ciprofloxacin.**

Q **Question 8.2 In a Patient undergoing Phacoemulsification, Intraoperatively you noted that Pieces do not Come to the Port.**

There is possibly a **posterior capsular rupture.** I will stop to assess and look for signs of capsular rupture. Signs suggestive of capsular rupture include **poor flowability, unstable anterior chamber, direct visualization of the edge of the rupture, direct visualization of vitreous in the anterior chamber, fragments falling away,** as well as **pupil snap sign** (for hydrorupture).

Q **Question 8.3 What are the Risk Factors for PCR?**

Factors can be divided into **patient factors, ocular factors,** and **intraoperative factors.** Patient factors include **uncooperative or moving patients, coughing, causes of increased vitreous pressure** such as **chronic obstructive lung disease,** and **obstructive sleep apnea.** Ocular factors include **small pupil (IA under iris), white cataract (higher risk of run-out), brunescent cataracts (loose floopy bag), high myopia (floppy bag), pseudoexfoliation syndrome, posterior polar cataract,** and **glaucoma (shallow AC, PC near).** Intraoperative factors include **high vitreous pressure after regional anesthesia, small capsulorrhexis, wound leak, unstable anterior chamber, inappropriate phacoemulsification settings,** and **poor lighting,** as well as **machine failure.**

Q **Question 8.4 How would you Manage Posterior Capsular Rupture?**

Principles of management include **early recognition, limiting the size of rupture, minimizing vitreous loss, safe removal of nuclear fragments, avoiding drop and implantation of appropriate intraocular lens.** It depends on the **stage of surgery, amount of vitreous loss,** and **size of remaining nuclear fragments.** Upon identifying the rupture, I will stop and inject viscoelastic through the side port over the rupture side and under the lens fragments to tamponade the vitreous, simultaneously turning off the infusion before removal of the phaco probe. I will assess the situation and look for vitreous loss. **If the fragments are small, I will extend the wound and insert a sheet's glide and phaco over it. If the fragments are large, I can attempt expression using viscoelastic or converting into an extracapsular cataract extraction with removal using the pediatric Vectis.** After that, I will perform a **thorough anterior vitrectomy** (bimanual or co-axial) and manual aspiration of the soft lens material.

My choice of intraocular lens implant will depend on the **anterior capsular support** and **size of the rupture**. If the rupture is small, I can implant a single-piece lens into the bag. If the rupture is large and anterior support is intact, I will implant a three-piece lens into the sulcus with posterior optic capture. If the anterior support is deficient, I can either insert an anterior chamber intraocular lens or leave the patient aphakic (need PI and anterior vitrectomy) for subsequent secondary posterior intraocular lens fixation. I will then close the wound with 10/0 nylon aiming for watertight closure, inject carbechol to miose the pupil, and check the wound and anterior chamber for vitreous. I will then inject subconjunctival steroids and antibiotics in the absence of contraindications, start the patient on pressure lowering medications (topical glaucoma drops and systemic oral acetazolamide), topical antibiotics and steroids, and **oral ciprofloxacin 500 mg twice a day.**

> **Q** **Question 8.5 What Complications will you Monitor for in Posterior Capsular Rupture?**

I will monitor the patient in the **early postoperative period for wound leak, hypotony, or increased intraocular pressure** as well as **endophthalmitis, suprachoroidal hemorrhage** or **choroidal effusion, retinal tears,** or **detachments**. In the **late postoperative period I will monitor for cystoid macular edema, persistent inflammation, retinal tears or detachments,** and **corneal decompensation.**

Management of PCR
- stage of surgery
- size of PCR
- presence of vitreous loss

Principles
- minimizing extention of PCR
- safe removal of nucleus
- minimizing vitreous loss
- implantation of appropriate lens

	Settings for Venturi System			Ant Vitrect
	Sculpting	Segment Removal	Epinucleus Removal	Cut Rate
Power (%)	30	20–30	10–15	400–600
Vacuum (mmhg)	30	300	150	150–200
Bottle ht (cm)	100	120	120	50

Q **Question 9.1 Viva Stem: What Issues do you need to Consider in Patients with Diabetes undergoing a Cataract Operation?**

In patients with diabetes, considerations include **visual potential, poorly dilating pupil, presence of neovascular glaucoma, presence and progression of diabetic retinopathy or macular edema, poor wound healing,** and **increased risk of infection.**

Preop: diabetes control, control retinopathy and macular edema, IOP control in neovascular glaucoma, manage poorly dilating pupil

Intraop: poorly dilated pupil, floppy iris syndrome, IOP

Postop: endophthalmitis, macular edema, raised IOP, diabetic retinopathy progression

Note: wounds might need to be sutured (PRP requires lens with inadvertant compression), large optic lens, insert acrylic lens/heparin coated

Q **Question 9.2 How would you Treat the Patient with Diabetes and Cataract?**

Treatment of a patient with diabetes and cataract can be divided into systemic and ocular. Systemically, I will co-manage with an internist to **ensure good glycemic control**. Ocular management can be divided into preoperative, intraoperative, and postoperative stages. Preoperatively, I will ensure that retinopathy and macular edema are controlled, perform **retinal photocoagulation if required, assess the visual potential** (might require FFA if mac ischaemia is suspected), and carry out **topical application of atropine** for poorly dilating pupils. Intraoperatively, I will perform the surgery under regional anesthesia (especially if pupil is small) sterile conditions and informed consent, implant a large optic lens, manage the **poorly dilating pupil, avoiding anterior chamber lens or silicone lenses,** and **suturing the wound.** Postoperatively, I will **monitor for infection** and **early dilation to assess retinopathy status** (at about the 2nd postoperative week), **control inflammation,** and **monitor for glaucoma.**

Q Question 10 Viva Stem: How would you Manage this Cataract (see Figures 1.3A and 1.3B) and what are the Issues Associated with It?

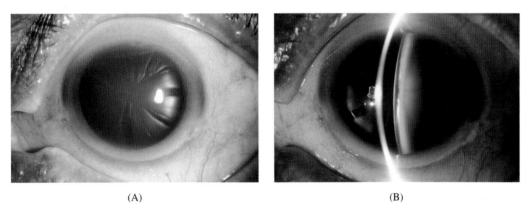

(A)   (B)

Figure 1.3 (A) Diffuse illumination of a brunescent cataract. (B) Slit beam examination of the brunescent cataract.

The photographs show the anterior segment of the right eye with a brunescent cataract. The pupil is widely dilated, there is no obvious subluxation of the lens, and the cornea is clear.

Issues and management can be divided into preoperative, intraoperative, and postoperative stages. Preoperatively, I will need to assess the visual potential using **relative afferent pupillary defect** and light projection if visual acuity is limited to hand movement or worse. If there is no view of the fundus, I will need to perform a **B scan.** Accurate biometry will be difficult as well. I will counsel the patient on the **guarded prognosis**, obtain **anterior chamber intraocular lens biometry**, have a **standby anterior vitrectomy**, and perform an **endothelial cell count** and **ultrasound biomicroscopy looking for zonulysis** (manage glaucoma if present due to subluxation). Intraoperatively, I will perform the surgery under informed consent regional anesthesia sterile conditions. Issues include poor red reflex and visualization of anterior capsule, increased risk of zonulysis and posterior capsular rupture (large floppy bag), corneal edema and wound burn, as well as tumbling of nuclear fragments. I will **stain the anterior capsule** with **vision blue**, ensure good hydrodissection, perform phacoemulsification using an *in situ* **chop technique** with a sharp second instrument, avoiding excessive manipulation to reduce zonular stress, **increase power and vacuum settings** to avoid rocking of the nucleus and chattering, respectively, **fill the anterior chamber with cohesive and dispersive viscoelastic (soft shell technique)** and **phaco in the pupil plane**, and **minimize tumbling, reducing settings at the last fragment to minimize surge risk**. Postoperatively, I will monitor for development of corneal decompensation and treat accordingly.

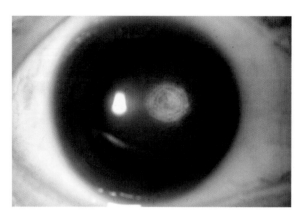

Figure 1.4 Posterior polar cataract.

The photograph shows the anterior segment of the right eye with a poster polar cataract with minimal nuclear sclerotic cataract.

Management of posterior polar cataract can be divided into preoperative, intraoperative, and postoperative stages.

Preoperatively, I will assess the visual function by checking the visual acuity and relative afferent pupillary defect, and conduct a dilated fundal examination. If the fundal view is poor, I will perform **a B scan.** I will counsel the patient regarding increased risk of complications especially posterior capsular rupture and have a **standby anterior vitrectomy and sulcus lens/anterior chamber intraocular lens biometry.**

Intraoperatively, I will perform the surgery under informed consent in the operating theater under regional anesthesia sterile conditions. After creating an adequately sized capsulorrhexis, I will perform **hydrodelamination** and **phacoemulsification of the nucleus under reduced parameters**. I will then proceed to remove the **epinucleus via a delamination technique,** taking care to ensure anterior chamber stability and to **inject viscoelastic prior to removal of instruments** (treat as per PCR — area is thinned out and removal of instruments with AC decompression can cause a rupture). After removal of the base, I will inspect carefully for posterior capsular rupture and manage accordingly, and finally I will implant the appropriate intraocular lens. If there is a posterior capsular rupture, postoperatively, I will monitor closely for **prolonged inflammation, raised intraocular pressure, cystoid macular edema, retinal tear/detachment,** and **endophthalmitis.**

Q **Question 12 Viva Stem: How would you Manage this Cataract (see Figure 1.5) and what are the Issues Associated with It?**

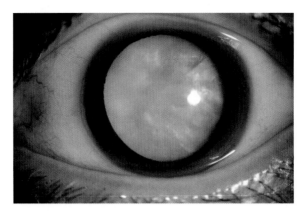

Figure 1.5 White cataract with areas of cystic cleft.

The photograph shows the anterior segment of the left eye with a white cataract with areas of fluid clefts and a clear cornea. The pupil is well dilated with no evidence of subluxation of the lens. I will cast a slit to examine the anterior chamber depth, look for anterior chamber activity, and measure the intraocular pressure.

Management of a white cataract can be divided into preoperative, intraoperative, and postoperative stages.

Preoperatively, I will assess the visual function by checking the visual acuity and relative afferent pupillary defect, and perform **a B scan**. I will counsel the patient regarding the increased risk of complications, especially posterior capsular rupture, and have on standby an **anterior vitrectomy** and a **sulcus lens/ACIOL biometry.**

Intraoperatively, I will perform the surgery under informed consent in the operating theater under regional anesthesia sterile conditions. If the anterior chamber is shallow, I will create a **longer more anteriorly placed** clear corneal incision followed by **staining of the capsule with vision blue under air**. I will inject adequate viscoelastic followed by **decompression of the bag** using a 27-gauge needle mounted on a 5-ml syringe. I will then initiate the capsulorrhexis with the needle, starting small and gradually enlarging (no need for subsequent hydrodissection). I will perform the phacoemulsification and aspiration of the liquefied cortex carefully, keeping in mind that the posterior capsule might be close.

Postoperatively, I will monitor for prolonged inflammation, glaucoma, and posterior capsular opacification.

Q **Question 13** OSCE Stem: Examine a Patient with the Anterior Segment Findings shown in Figure 1.6.

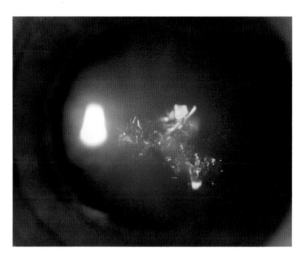

Figure 1.6 Christmas tree cataract secondary to myotonia dystrophica.

On general examination of the patient, I find that the patient has an **expressionless Hatchet facies** with **frontal balding, temporalis** and **masseter wasting with bilateral ptosis.** On examination of the right eye, the most obvious abnormality is the presence of **crystalline opacities in the lens suggestive of a Christmas tree cataract.** The anterior chamber is otherwise deep and quiet and the cornea is clear. It is not associated with microphthalmos. Examination of the fellow eye shows similar findings. I will check the visual acuity, examine **the pupils for light near dissociation** and **extraocular movements for limitation,** check the intraocular pressure for **hypotonia** (associated with ciliary body detachment), and perform a dilated fundal examination for maculopathy and pigmentary retinopathy, as well as assess for myotonic grip. I will also examine the family members. This patient has Christmas tree cataract associated with myotonic dystorphica.

Q **Question 14** Viva Stem: How would you Perform Sclera Fixation of an Intraocular Lens?

I will perform the procedure under informed consent in the operating theater with general anesthesia under sterile conditions. I will create two **Hoffman pockets,** one at **8 o'clock** and the other at **2 o'clock**. I will then create a 6-mm superior **limbal incision** and perform an adequate **anterior vitrectomy**. I will pass a **9/0 single armed prolene suture on a long**

straight needle through the Hoffman pocket (full thickness) at 2 o'clock, **1.5 mm posterior to the limbus,** into the sulcus region, advancing parallel to the iris plane. The tip of the needle will then be **received by a 25G needle** entered from the 8 o'clock position and subsequently **externalized.** Two sutures will be passed through in this manner. I will externalize the sutures passing across the pupil through the limbal incision using Kuglan hooks, cut it and tie it onto the haptics of a **three-piece intraocular lens** to achieve a **two-point fixation** on each haptic. I will then insert the intraocular lens through the limbal incision (if the IOL is folded and introduced, a smaller limbal incision would suffice) and place it under the iris. The sutures at each end are pulled through under the sclera pocket roof, and subsequently tied with the **knots under the sclera pocket roof** and the **tension adjusted to ensure good lens centration**. I will then create a surgical iridectomy prior to closure of the limbal wound.

CHAPTER 2

CORNEA

Q **Question 1.1 OSCE Stem: Anterior Segment Examination of the following Patient (see Figures 2.1A and 2.1B).**

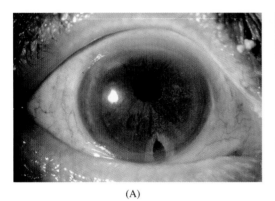
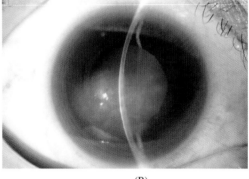

(A) (B)

Figure 2.1 (A) Left Fuch's endothelial corneal dystrophy post Descemet Stripping Automated Endothelial Keratoplasty with an inferior Ando peripheral iridectomy. (B) Right eye of the same patient with bullous keratopathy secondary to FECD. The patient will need DSAEK in this eye as well.

On examination of the left eye, there is presence of an endothelial **lamellar keratoplasty** with four **venting incisions**. The graft is attached **clear** and well-centered with **no evidence of corneal decompensation** or **rejection**. The anterior chamber is deep and **quiet** without keratic precipitates. There is presence of an **inferior Ando peripheral iridectomy** and the patient has a posterior chamber intraocular lens. There are **no laser peripheral iridotomy, glaucoma filtration surgery,** or **glaucoma drainage devices**. On examination of the right eye, there are multiple **central guttata** seen with associated **corneal edema** and **bullous keratopathy involving the visual axis but no stromal scarring**. The anterior chamber is deep and quiet and the patient is phakic with a nuclear sclerotic cataract. There is absence of **laser peripheral iridotomy, glaucoma filtration surgery,** and **glaucoma drainage device**. This patient has **bilateral corneal decompensation likely secondary to Fuch's endothelial dystrophy**, and the right is stable post endothelial keratoplasty. I will check the visual acuity, relative afferent pupillary defect, and intraocular pressure, and perform a dilated fundal examination for increased cup disc ratio and any retina or macula pathologies that might affect visual potential. I will examine the family members. I will also check the **endothelial cell count** and **the pachymetry**.

> **Q** **Question 1.2** What are the Factors Affecting your Management of Patients with FED and Cataract?

The management of patients with FED and cataract can be challenging, and depends on the **visual prognosis**; it will require treatment for both the cornea and the cataract. Indications for optical keratoplasty include **blurring of vision in the morning, severe edema on clinical examination, central corneal thickness more than 650 microns, endothelial cell count less than 800,** and **diurnal variation of corneal thickness by more than 10%**. If the cataract is visually significant, I will perform a cataract extraction for the patient. If there is significant corneal decompensation with the cataract, I will perform a triple procedure of combined cataract extraction and intraocular lens implant with optical keratoplasty.

In this patient, if visual prognosis is good, I will offer a combined **triple procedure —** keratoplasty with cataract extraction and intraocular lens implant versus **staged cataract extraction followed by keratoplasty**. In this patient, there is minimal stromal scarring, and he is suitable for either **full-thickness penetrating keratoplasty** or **lamellar descemet's stripping automated endothelial keratoplasty**. (If there is significant scarring, PK should be performed.)

> **Q** **Question 1.3** What are the Difficulties between Combined and Non-Combined Procedures?

In both procedures, obtaining **accurate biometry is difficult** and **intraocular visualization is poor**. There is a **higher risk of complications** such as posterior capsular rupture. In a triple procedure, the patient only undergoes a single operation with reduced costs. In a staged procedure, the patient has to undergo two operations with the advantage of delaying the cornea graft procedure.

- Advantages of staged procedure: IOL stability in the bag, easier to manage if complications occur, delay of graft procedure
- Advantages of combined procedure: faster visual recovery, reduced number of operations

Q Question 1.4 Picture of Endothelial Cell Count.

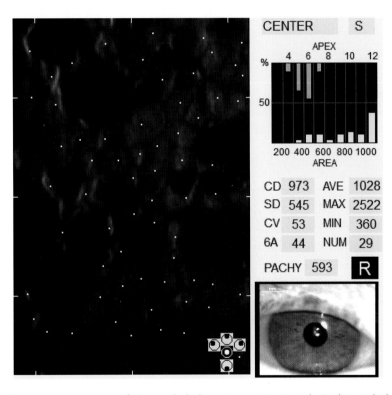

Figure 2.2 Specular microscopy of the endothelium in a patient with Fuch's endothelial corneal dystrophy.

This is the **specular microscopy** of the patient's right eye. There is reduced **cellular density** with 973 cells per mm^2. The **coefficient of variation** is raised at 53 and **hexagonality** (6A) is reduced at 44%. The **average cell volume is increased** and the **total number of cells counted** is 29. **Corneal thickness** is increased at 593 microns. There is graphical evidence of **pleomorphism** and **polymeganthism** as evidenced by the increased spread of the graph. On the pictorial scale, there are **areas of guttata** seen with **loss of hexagonality** of the cells and **variation of cell sizes**. (Ideal figures: NUM $\geq$ 100, CV < 40, 6A $\geq$ 60, CD is age-dependent.)

Q **Question 2.1 OSCE Stem: Anterior Segment Examination of the following Patient.**

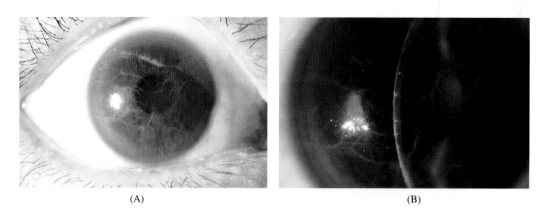

(A)   (B)

Figures 2.3A and 2.3B The diffuse and slit beam photos demonstrate the signs seen in a patient with lattice dystrophy. Note that the linear branching opacities are mainly located in the anterior to mid-stroma and has clear intervening spaces

On examination of the anterior segment, there are **linear rope-like branching opacities** in the **mid-stroma** involving the **visual axis extending toward the periphery but sparing the limbus** with **clear intervening spaces**. The anterior chamber is deep and quiet and the patient is phakic. I will check the contralateral eye. I will **check the visual acuity** and **corneal sensation, examine the family members, stain the cornea for epithelial defects**, and **examine the patient's history for recurrent corneal erosions**. I will check systemically for features of **Meretoja syndrome** such as **cutis laxa, myopathicfacies, facial nerve palsy (CN7)**, and **long pendulous ears**. In summary, this patient has **lattice dystrophy**. Management would depend on the visual acuity and ocular symptoms. If there is ocular pain secondary to recurrent corneal erosions, I will treat with antibiotic cover and copious lubricants, and keep in view tetracyclines and bandage contact lens. If there is frequent recurrence, anterior stromal micropuncture or phototherapeutic keratectomy can be considered. If visual acuity is poor, I will consider **lamellar keratoplasty** for the patient.

Q **Question 2.2 Describe the Histopathological Slide shown below.**

This is the histological slide through the corneal stroma. The most significant abnormality is the presence of **irregular eosinophilic deposits within the anterior stroma, suggestive of amyloid deposits**. The overlying **epithelium is otherwise intact**.

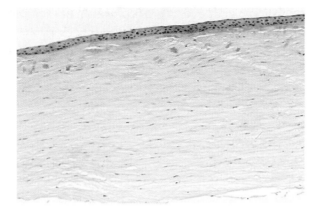

Figure 2.4 Lattice corneal dystrophy. Note the small irregular deposits of eosinophilic material (amyloid) in the superficial corneal stroma (hematoxylin and eosin stain, original magnification x60).

Q **Question 2.3 What is the Inheritance?**

Autosomal dominant, TGFβ1 gene, 5_q31 chromosome

Q **Question 3 OSCE Stem: Examination of Patient (see Figures 2.5A and 2.5B), starting with the Left Eye.**

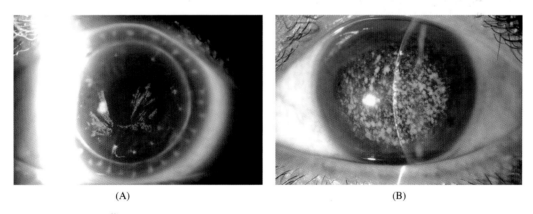

(A) (B)

Figure 2.5 (A) The sclerotic scatter highlights the recurrence of granular dystrophy within a deep anterior lamellar graft, close to but not involving the visual axis. (B) This photo of the contralateral eye of the same patient shows extensive granular deposits within the stroma obscuring the visual axis. Vision is poor in this eye unless the patient undergoes a transplant.

On examination of the patient's left eye, there is presence of multiple **breadcrumb-like** deposits within the **mid-stroma** with **clear intervening spaces** involving the central visual axis and extending to but **not involving the limbus**. Peripherally the cornea is clear. There are no obvious epithelial defects. The anterior chamber is deep and quiet with a mild nuclear sclerotic cataract. On examination of the right eye, there is presence of a corneal graft with multiple **interrupted sutures** which have since been removed. On casting a slit at the graft host junction, there is a **clear interface suggesting that this is a deep anterior lamellar keratoplasty**. There are whitish streaks of opacities within the mid stroma of the graft inferiorly extending upward to involve the visual axis with clear intervening spaces. There is no epithelial defect, **no features of corneal rejection** such as corneal edema and keratic precipitates. The anterior chamber is deep and quiet with a mild nuclear sclerotic cataract. There are no glaucoma filtration surgery or drainage device implantation. This patient likely has **bilateral granular dystrophy** status post **right deep anterior lamellar keratoplasty** with evidence of **recurrence**. I will check the visual acuity and intraocular pressure. I will stain the cornea and examine the disc especially of the right eye (for steroid induced glaucoma). I will examine the patient's history for recurrent corneal erosions and examine the parents of the patient.

Q **Question 4 OSCE Stem: Examination of a Patient (see Figures 2.6A and 2.6B).**

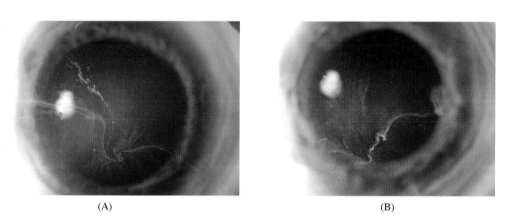

(A)   (B)

Figures 2.6A and 2.6B   Bilateral vortex keratopathy secondary to amiodarone.

On examination of the anterior segment, there are features of **vortex keratopathy** as evidenced by **brownish pigment deposits on the epithelium in a whorl-like pattern** involving the visual axis. Otherwise the cornea is **clear with no evidence of crystalline keratopathy**. There are **no tortuous conjunctival vessels that might suggest underlying Fabry's disease**. The anterior chamber is deep and quiet and there is no significant cataract. I will examine the fundus for disc swelling and atrophy (tamoxifen), crystalline retinopathy (tamoxifen), bull's eye maculopathy (chlorpromazine, hydroxychloroquine, tamoxifen, clofazimine), and macular edema (tamoxifen) and pseudo retinitis pigmentosa changes (suggestive of chlorpromazine or hydroxychloroquine). I will examine systemically for **angiokeratomas** and **rheumatoid arthritis**, check the cardiovascular system pulse rate and electrocardiogram for **arrhythmias**, and examine the patient's history for **indomethacin use for arthritis, tamoxifen use for breast cancer, amiodarone and hydroxychloroquine use**, and **chlorpromazine use for psychosis/depression**.

Note:
Drugs for crystalline retinopathy — tamoxifen/talcosis/canthaxanthin/methoxyflurane/nitrofurantoin
Drugs for bull's eye maculopathy — tamoxifen/hydroxychloroquine/chlorquine/clofazimine

> **Q** **Question 5.1 Viva Stem: How do you Manage a Patient with the Condition shown in Figure 2.7?**

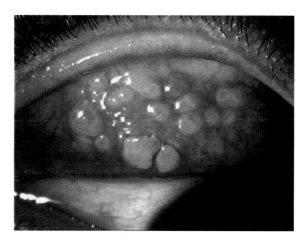

Figure 2.7   Giant papillae in a patient with vernal keratoconjunctivitis.

This is the limited anterior segment photograph showing large **cobblestone papillae** of the upper tarsal conjunctiva. The conjunctiva appears otherwise mildly injected and the cornea appears clear. The patient is likely to have **atopic keratoconjunctivitis/vernal keratoconjunctivitis**. I will check the visual acuity, relative afferent papillary defect, and intraocular pressures (for steroid-induced glaucoma), and check the rest of the cornea for complications such as **shield ulcer** and **keratoconus**. I will check the limbus **for pseudogerontoxon** and **Horner's trantas** dots, examine the lens for **cataract** (especially ASC) and phacodonesis, and perform a dilated fundal examination for **increased cup-disc ratio**, **retinal tears**, and **detachment**. I will examine the fellow eye, check the **refractive status**, and examine systemically for features of atopy. I will examine the patient's history for duration and symptoms, any itch/pain/blurring of vision, frequency of rubbing, exposure, any contact lens use, and associated atopic conditions such as eczema, allergic rhinitis, and asthma.

Q Question 5.2 What is the Difference between Vernal Keratoconjunctivitis (VKC) and Atopic Keratoconjunctivitis (AKC)?

VKC occurs in **younger children** and **predominantly males** with greater involvement of the **superior tarsal conjunctiva** compared to inferior tarsal conjunctiva. There is **greater incidence of shield ulcers but a better visual prognosis**. AKC occurs in older children with no gender predilection, who have greater involvement of inferior tarsal conjunctiva, and who have reduced incidence of shield ulcers but a poorer visual prognosis.

Q Question 5.3 How would you Manage.

Principles of management include **avoidance of allergens, lubrication, treatment of allergy and inflammation, treatment of associated complications**, and **visual rehabilitation**. Management can be divided into **systemic** and **ocular**. I will refer to the internist for management of systemic atopy. Ocular treatment involves preservative free lubricants, anti-histamines and mast cell stabilizers, topical steroids during episodes of flare, steroid-sparing agents if required (e.g. CSA 0.05% or tacrolimus drops), failing which oral steroids will have to be considered. I will monitor for the development of shield ulcers, amblyopia (if the patient is a child), keratoconus, cataracts, glaucoma secondary to steroid use, and retinal tears or detachment. Uncontrolled cases might need supratarsal steroid injection or papillectomy. Shield ulcers not responsive to medical therapy might need debridement/superficial keratectomy with amniotic membrane transplant.

Q Question 6.1 Viva Stem: Patient presenting with Acute Pain and Blurring of Vision over the past three days (see Figure 2.8).

This is a colour photograph of the patient's right eye with a **large central infiltrate obscuring the visual axis** with associated overlying subtotal epithelial defect, diffuse injection, and **hypopyon**. View of the anterior chamber is poor but **appears to be formed**. I will check the visual acuity and relative afferent pupillary defect by the reverse method, check for thinning and intraocular pressure, and **perform a B scan for vitritis**. I will take the patient's history for any **trauma** and **contact lens use**, as well as for **immunocompromised state/immunosuppressive medications**.

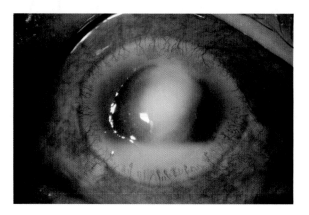

Figure 2.8 This patient has a long history of contact lens use and has developed contact lens-related infective keratitis with reactive hypopyon.

Q Question 6.2 How would you Manage a Patient who is a Contact Lens user, and whose Vitreous is Clear on a B Scan?

I will explain to the patient the **guarded prognosis**, advice the patient to **stop contact lens use** immediately in both eyes, and **admit the patient**. I will scrape the border of the infiltrate avoiding areas of thinning, **sending off for gram stain and cultures** (blood, choc agar, BHIB, thioglycate, sabourad's), start the patient on **intensive hourly fortified broad-spectrum antibiotics** in the absence of contraindications, and **review daily with serial B scans**.

Q Question 6.3 How do you Monitor the Patient in Question 6.2 for Improvement?

I will look for the following: (1) symptoms (subjective) such as reduction in pain and photophobia and improvement of visual acuity, and (2) signs (objective) such as consolidation of infiltrate, reduction in anterior chamber activity, reduction in size of infiltrate and epithelial defect, reduction of corneal haze, and improvement in vision.

Q **Question 6.4** **What is the Indication for a Corneal Biopsy and how do you Perform It?**

Corneal biopsy is indicated in the patient if the **infective keratitis is not responding to treatment with negative cultures**. I will stop the antibiotics **24 hours** prior and perform the surgery under informed consent in the operating theater under regional anesthesia and sterile conditions with a **tectonic graft on standby**. I will use a **2-mm dermatological trephine**, choosing a site **away from the visual axis incorporating both the normal cornea and the edge and base of the ulcer, avoiding areas of thinning**, then perform a **partial-thickness trephination**, and finally complete the **lamellar dissection with a crescent blade**. I will **cut the biopsy into quadrants** and send these for **histology and culture studies** while restarting the patient on intensive antibiotic eye drops.

Note: Other indications: suspected malignancies.

Q **Question 6.5** **What are the Other Possible Methods of Identifying the Organism?**

Other possible methods include **polymerase chain reaction** and **confocal microscopy**.

Note: Another possible question could be: If the initial scrapping is negative and is not responding to treatment, what can you do?

I can stop the treatment for 24 hours and rescrape the lesion (**consider sending for fungal** and **acanthemeba**); if that is negative, I will then stop treatment for 24 hours and perform a corneal biopsy. Other modalities include **polymerase chain reaction** or **confocal microscopy**.

Q **Question 7.1** **Viva Stem: How would you Perform a Corneal Glue Procedure?**

I will perform corneal gluing (cyanoacrylate) for **corneal perforation < 2 mm**. I will perform the procedure under informed consent in the operating theater under general anesthesia **avoiding depolarizing agents**. Clean and drape with **chlorhexidine**, opening the lids with **lid traction sutures** or **Jeffrey's lid retractor**, taking **swabs for microscopy and cultures**. I will reform the **anterior chamber via an anterior chamber paracentesis** and **reposit viable tissue**. I will then **dry and debride** the area of perforation. I will punch out a small **3-mm sterile plastic disc** using dermatological trephine, **attach it to an orange stick with fucithalmic**, apply **cyanoacrylate (tissue glue) onto the disc**, and **apply it to the perforated site** and irrigate. Once the glue has set, I will remove the stick, **check for wound leak using fluorescein, place a bandage contact lens** over the site, and restart the patient on antibiotic eye drops.

Question 7.2 What are the Indications and Contraindications for the Corneal Glue Procedure?

The indications for corneal glue are for perforations **less than 2mm, no tissue prolapse, formed anterior chamber, no tissue or vitreous loss, no infection**. The procedure is to augment suture closure of corneal lacerations with small residual leak and is suitable for patients who are not fit for surgery. Contraindications include perforations more than 2mm, presence of infection, or uveal prolapse.

Question 8.1 OSCE Stem: Examination of Patient with the Findings shown in Figure 2.9.

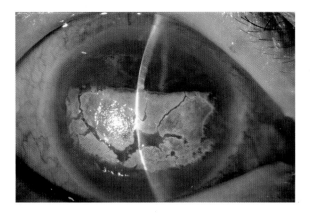

Figure 2.9 This patient has had a longstanding history of primary angle closure glaucoma on multiple glaucoma medications. The cornea has developed band keratopathy and is decompensating from persistently raised intraocular medications. Visual prognosis is poor.

This is the anterior segment photograph of the patient's right eye showing the presence of **subepithelial calcium deposits** with a **Swiss-cheese appearance** suggestive of band keratopathy extending horizontally from 9 to 3 o'clock in the **interpalpebral region** obscuring the visual axis with associated corneal edema and hazy view of the anterior chamber. There is presence of a **superior temporal peripheral iridotomy** (not well seen in this photograph) but no glaucoma filtration surgery or drainage device. There is no inferior Ando peripheral iridectomy and no keratic precipitates (look for clues to other causes of band K). On examination of the contralateral eye, the anterior chamber is shallow with a patent superior temporal peripheral iridotomy. The patient likely has **right chronic angle closure glaucoma with corneal decompensation and band keratopathy**. I will check the visual acuity and relative afferent papillary defect by the reverse method, and perform a dilated fundal examination for increased cup-disc ratio. If the view is poor, I will perform a B scan and examine the patient's medication history and see if the patient has had previous acute angle closure attacks. (If there are no obvious causes found, I will examine the patient's history for systemic conditions like renal failure.)

Q **Question 8.2 How do you Treat Band Keratopathy?**

Treatment depends on symptoms as well as whether the band keratopathy involves the visual axis in a patient with good visual prognosis. If the patient is **symptomatic or it involves the visual axis**, I will perform chelation under informed consent in the operating theater under topical anesthesia in sterile conditions. I will first scrape off the overlying epithelium using a pterygium blade and soak the area of band keratopathy with **3% ethylene-diamine-tetraacetic acid for three to five minutes** before **scraping off the band keratopathy using a pterygium blade**. I will then inject subconjunctival antibiotics and steroids and place a bandage contact lens over the site.

Causes of Band Keratopathy	
Systemic	**Ocular**
• Hypercalcemia	• Chronic cornea edema
• Hyperparathyroidism	• Long standing poor ocular surface
• Renal failure	• SO in AC
• Hyperurecemia	• Chronic uveitis
	• Glaucoma

Q **Question 9 Viva Stem: How would you Manage a Patient Hit by a Wooden Branch and Presents with Pain and Blurring of Vision (see Figure 2.10)?**

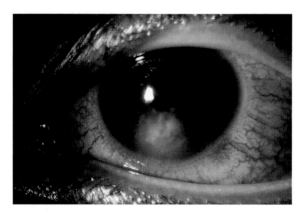

Figure 2.10   The ulcer has a whitish feathery appearance with satellite lesions. This is suggestive of a fungal keratitis in the context of trauma involving vegetative material.

This is the anterior segment photograph of the patient's left eye. There is an area of **whitish infiltrate** measuring about one-third the diameter of the cornea **inferior to the visual axis** with irregular **feathery edges** and **satellite lesions** along the superior edge together with conjunctival injection. I will cast a slit to assess the depth of the involvement. The rest of the cornea is quite clear with **absence of ground glass haze** and immune ring. I will check the visual acuity, anterior chamber activity, and intraocular pressure, and perform a dilated fundal examination for posterior involvement. I will also check the fellow eye and examine the patient's history for **trauma associated with vegetative material, immunocompromised states**, or **use of immunosuppressive medications**. This patient likely has atypical infective keratitis secondary to fungal infection.

Features of fungal keratitis include an **indolent course, greyish white elevated infiltrate, feathery indistinct borders, satellite lesions, endothelial plaque**, and **ring infiltrate**.

Fungal keratitis is a **potential blinding disease** and requires immediate treatment. Treatment is **difficult and can be prolonged**; the patient might need **multiple drugs** and **require surgical intervention**. I will examine the patient's history for **trauma, vegetative material entry**, and **immunosuppression**. I will scrape the **lesion for cultures and microscopy**, admit the patient and start the patient on topical **anti-fungal therapy with antibiotic cover** in the absence of contraindications. I will consider **oral anti-fungals** if the lesion is large and involves the limbus, and if there is the presence of hypopyon or evidence of intraocular penetration. Medications can be divided into **fungicidal** and **fungistatic**. **Fungicidal drugs include polyenes such as natamycin for filamentous fungi and amphotericin for non filamentous fungi. Fungistatic drugs include imidazoles** such as **voriconazole** and **ketoconazole**. I will review the patient daily and **debride the cornea epithelium to enhance penetration of the anti-fungal eye drops**, and **monitor for thinning, raised intr-ocular pressure**, and **endophthalmitis**. If infection is progressing or not responsive to treatment, I will consider rescraping, performing confocal microscopy or corneal biopsy, and performing intrastromal injection of amphotericin or voriconazole. If these fail, a **therapeutic keratoplasty** might then be required (but carries a poor prognosis).

Note: Differentials to atypical keratitis: fungal, acanthemeba, Norcardia, mycobacterium/atypical mycobacterium. In the Singapore National Eye Centre, we usually use a combination of natamycin and amphotericin.

Other presentation of atypical infective keratitis (see Fig. 2.11).

Q Question 10.1 Viva Stem: How would you Manage a 30-Year-old Patient with the following Presentation (see Figure 2.12)?

This is the limited anterior segment photograph of the left eye showing a **dendritic ulcer with dichotomous branching and terminal bulbs**. The rest of the cornea appears. There

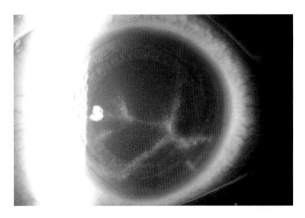

Figure 2.11 This is another presentation of atypical infective keratitis. The perineural infiltrates are well highlighted by the sclerotic scatter technique in this photograph. This patient has acanthamoeba infective keratitis.

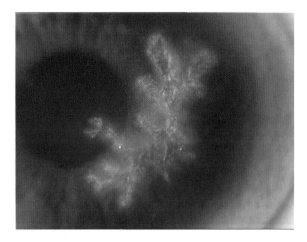

Figure 2.12 HSV dendrite — classical configuration of dichotomous branching with terminal bulbs.

are no obvious areas of **posterior** or **peripheral anterior synaechia** and **keratic precipitates** but I would examine the whole eye. This patient has **herpes simplex virus keratitis**. I will first examine the patient's history for duration of symptoms, progression, and possible immunocompromised state and previous vesicular rash. I will then check the visual acuity and relative afferent pupillary defect, assess the lesion, check the **corneal sensation** and intraocular pressure, assess the anterior chamber for keratitic precipitates and cellular activity, perform a dilated fundal examination for **vasculitis** and **acute retinal necrosis**, and **examine systemically for vesicular rash**. In view of the epithelial keratitis, I will first treat with **topical broad-spectrum preservative-free antibiotics**, copious amount of **preservative free lubricants**, and **topical 3% acyclovir ointment five times a day**. If there is anterior segment activity, **I will treat with oral acyclovir 400 mg five times per**

day in view of the anterior chamber activity (5% ointment five times per day to rash if there is). If the patient develops stromal keratitis, **I will start the patient on preservative-free topical steroids once the epithelium has healed**. I will investigate this patient, checking for retroviral infection and carry out a liver function test for suitability of oral acyclovir.

Q Question 10.2 Discuss the Herpetic Eye Disease Study.

The herpetic eye disease study (HEDS) is a **multicenter randomized control study** divided into two parts. The first study showed that in patients receiving topical anti-virals, steroid eye drops improved visual outcomes and reduced severity in stromal keratitis. Addition of oral anti-virals did not confer any benefits. Treatment of anterior uveitis, though not statistically significant, favored the use of oral acyclovir. The second study showed that oral anti-virals did not prevent progression from epithelial keratitis to stromal keratitis. Prophylactic dose of 400 mg twice a day oral acyclovir, in patients with at least two recurrences, for one year after resolution of acute episodes reduced recurrence of stromal keratitis.

HEDS	HEDS1:
	• Topical steroids: beneficial for stromal keratitis
	• PO acyclovir **400 mg 5x/day**
	1) no difference for stromal keratitis
	2) beneficial for uveitis
	HEDS2
	• PO acyclovir **400mg 2x/day** for recurrent stromal keratitis (≥ 2)
	1) decreases rate of recurrence
	2) does not prevent progression from epithelial to stromal

Q Question 11.1 Viva Stem: How do you Manage a 25-year-old Patient who Presents with Recurrent Eye Pain and Redness?

I will first need to look for sight-threatening causes. Sight-threatening causes can be divided into ocular and orbital causes. **Ocular causes include scleritis, glaucoma, uveitis, infective keratitis (contact lens-related), exposure keratitis, limbal stem cell deficiency,** and **optic neuritis. Orbital causes include thyroid eye disease, orbital inflammatory disease,** and **dacryoadenitis**. Other common causes include dry eyes, allergic conjunctivitis (more with itch), recurrent corneal erosions, episcleritis, and lid abnormalities like epiblepharon. I will examine the patient's history for onset and progression of the condition, blurring of vision, presence of diplopia, any previous trauma, contact lens use, pain on extraocular movements, any past medical history, any previous ocular surgery, and features of systemic inflammatory disease. I will examine the patient for visual acuity and relative afferent pupillary defect; check the extraocular movements; check for proptosis using Hertel's exophthalmometer; check anterior segment staining for corneal abrasions, abnormal lid or lash position, presence of infective keratitis or evidence of contact lens overuse, and features of limbal stem cell deficiency; check the anterior segment for keratatic precipitates and activity; check the intraocular pressure; and finally, perform a dilated fundal examination for vitritis and disc swelling.

Q Question 11.2 How would you Manage a Patient with Recurrent Corneal Erosion?

The causes of recurrent corneal erosion can be divided into **congenital** and **acquired** causes. Congenital causes include **corneal epithelial** and **stromal dystrophies**, as well as **congenital limbal stem cell deficiency such as aniridia and Riley Day syndrome**. **Acquired causes include post-trauma, contact lens use, exposure keratopathy, neurotropic, chemical injury, Steven Johnson syndrome, chronic use of topical medications** or **anaesthetic abuse**, and **lid abnormalities** such as **epiblepharon**. I will examine the patient's history for contact lens use, previous trauma, previous chemical injuries or Steven Johnson syndrome, checking the anterior segment for corneal dystrophies, lagophthalmos, Bell's reflex, and corneal sensation (DDX neurotropic/exposure keratopathy). Principles of management include **removal of any offending agent/treating underlying cause, treating any concurrent infection, supporting healing**, and **prevention of recurrence**. I will first stop any offending agent such as contact lens use, treat concurrent infection with topical preservative-free broad-spectrum antibiotics in the absence of contraindications, support healing by using copious amounts of topical preservative-free lubricants and ointment, place a bandage contact lens if there is no infection, start the patient on chlortetracycline ointment, oral vitamin C (+/–doxycycline as indicated), and consider **lateral tarrsoharphy** or **botulinium injections** for severe exposure keratopathy. To prevent recurrence, **continuation of lubricants can be used, failing which surgical therapy such as debridement, diamond burr, anterior stromal micropuncture**, and **phototherapeutic keratectomy can be considered**.

Q Question 12.1 OSCE Stem: Examine a Patient with the following Anterior Segment findings (see Figures 2.3A and 2.3B).

On examination of the anterior segment of the left eye, there is a large area of **stromal opacity** in the left eye extending from 3 toward 9 o'clock involving the visual axis with **stromal vascularization** and **ghost vessels** but **no salmon pink patch**. The remaining

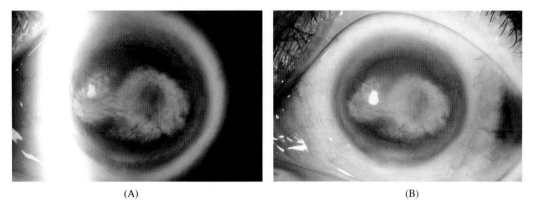

(A)	(B)

Figures 2.13A and 2.13B This patient has a dense left interstitial keratitis scar as a result of previous herpes simplex infection. Note the ghost vessels that are better seen with the sclerotic scatter technique.

cornea is clear, the conjunctiva is white, and there are **no old pigmented keratitic precipitates** and **no associated iris atrophy** or **iris nodules**. The anterior chamber view is **partially obstructed** but it is grossly deep and quiet with no posterior or peripheral anterior synaechiae. I will examine the other eye, checking the intraocular pressure and examining the fundus for **optic atrophy** and **salt and pepper retinopathy**. I will check the visual acuity, **corneal sensation**, and **pupils for Agryl Robertson pupil, examine systemically for saddle shape nose (congenital syphilis), notched incisors, deafness,** and **vertigo (Cogan's syndrome).**

Q Question 12.2 What are the Causes of Interstitial Keratitis?

The causes can be divided into **infective and non-infective** causes. Infective causes include viral causes such as herpes simplex, varicella zoster, bacterial causes such as tuberculosis, syphilis, leprosy, and Lyme disease. Non-infective causes include sarcoidosis and Cogan's disease.

Q Question 13.1 OSCE Stem: Examine a Patient with the following findings (see Figures 2.14A and 2.14B).

On examination of the right eye, there is **diffuse corneal edema** worse centrally with descemet membrane folds. There is associated bullae and microcystic edema. The anterior chamber is shallow with the presence of a **peripheral laser iridotomy superior nasally** that is **patent on retro-illumination**. Patient is phakic with a nuclear sclerotic cataract. Otherwise the eye is white with **absence of glaucoma filtration surgery or glaucoma**

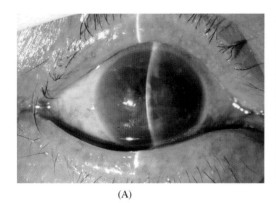
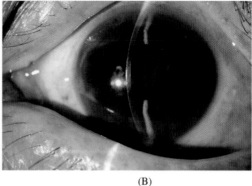

(A)   (B)

Figure 2.14 (A) Right corneal decompensation secondary to laser peripheral iridotomy in an eye that was previously diagnosed as a primary angle closure suspect. (B) Left primary angle closure suspect with prophylactic superior nasal laser peripheral iridotomy.

drainage device. On examination of the left eye, the cornea is clear with **no evidence of decompensation**. There is **no guttata** but the anterior chamber is **shallow** with a **superior nasal peripheral laser iridotomy** that is patent on retro-illumination. The eye is phakic with a nuclear sclerotic cataract and there is no glaucoma drainage device nor glaucoma filtration surgery. I will check the **visual acuity, relative afferent pupillary defect (by the reverse method if visualization of pupil is difficult), perform an indentational gonioscopy, check the intraocular pressure, conduct a dilated fundal examination for glaucomatous disc changes, and conduct a formal visual field assessment**. In summary, this patient has **bilateral laser peripheral iridotomy for primary angle closure disease spectrum** with **right corneal decompensation**. (Cause of the corneal decompensation could be secondary to APAC or LPI.)

Q **Question 13.2 What are the Common Causes of Bullous Keratopathy?**

The common causes of bullous keratopathy are **Fuch's endothelial dystrophy**, iatrogenic from laser peripheral iridotomy and **pseudophakic bullous keratopathy, traumatic, infective secondary to cytomegalovirus anterior uveitis**, and **uncontrolled glaucoma**.

Q **Question 13.3 How would you Manage a Patient with Moderate Bullous Keratopathy using Laser Peripheral Iridotomy?**

Management of bullous keratopathy can be challenging, and depends on the **underlying cause, visual prognosis**, and **ocular symptoms**. For this patient, I will check the cup-disc ratio and intraocular pressure and control them medically in the absence of contraindications in view of the peripheral iridotomy. If the prognosis is **poor** and the patient is **asymptomatic**, I will treat conservatively (with lubricants, hypertonic saline eye drops, and ointment, hair-dryer) and monitor the patient. If the patient is **symptomatic**, I will consider putting a band-age contact lens if there is no epithelial defect (as ED can be infected) with antibiotic cover, failing which I will then consider lateral tarsorrhaphy, botulinum injection to the eyelids (rubbing of bullae that causes pain), conjunctival flap procedure, retrobulbar alcohol injec-tion or evisceration/enucleation. If the visual prognosis is good, the patient will require optical keratoplasty (lamellar versus full thickness).

Q | **Question 14** Viva Stem: How will you Manage a Patient who Presents with Pain and Redness with Photophobia for one month (see Figure 2.15)?

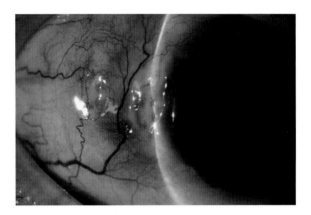

Figure 2.15

This is the anterior segment photo graph of the patient's right eye showing an injected eye temporally with **dilated deep scleral vessels**. Temporally at 9 o'clock, there is an area of scleral **thinning of about 50% exposing the underlying choroidal hue** but no calcified plaques or infiltrates. There is mild **peripheral ulcerative keratitis** of the adjacent periph-eral cornea which otherwise appears clear. This patient has **necrotizing anterior scler-okeratitis**. I will check the visual acuity, intraocular pressure, and anterior segment for keratitic precipitates, checking for activity as well as iris nodules. I will perform a dilated fundal examination to look for disc swelling, exudative retinal detachments, and vasculitis; assess the extraocular movements; and check for proptosis. I will perform a **gentle B scan to look for posterior scleritis** (fluid in subtenon space). I will examine the fellow eye as well, and **examine systemically for erythema of the ear, joint deformities**, and **saddle shape nose**. I will examine the patient's history for previous episodes and joint pains, rashes, and ear pain that might suggest a **systemic autoimmune condition**; examine the patient's contact history for tuberculosis and constitutional symptoms such as fever and weight loss; and examine the patient's sexual history. This is a sight-threatening condition and potentially life threatening (sclerokeratitis is associated with systemic conditions). Treatment can be divided into systemic and ocular. I will investigate by **swabbing the area of thinning** and send off for gram stains (microscopy) and cultures, performing investigations for the diagnosis and steroid workup. I will admit the patient and co-manage the patient with a rheumatologist systemically, and start the patient **on intravenous steroids and immunosuppression** in the absence of contraindications (as its likely systemic underlying condition). For the ocular management, I will need to treat the inflammation and prevent infection. I will refer to the corneal specialist and start the patient on copious amounts of **preservative-free lubricants, broad spectrum preservative-free antibiotics, cycloplegics, and intensive preservative-free steroid drops** (keep in mind that steroids might induce corneal melt). I will monitor the patient daily to assess for impending perforation, raised intraocular pressure, and exudative retinal detachment. If there is a risk of impending perforation, the patient will need surgical intervention (usually tectonic graft using donor sclera, cornea, fascia lata, dermis, or periosteum.)

Investigations: FBC ESR CRP UECr c-ANCA p-ANCA ANA RF anti-dsDNA CXR mantoux T spot/TB quantiferon syphilis LIA IgG and IgM VDRL conjunctival swabs for concomitant infections. For steroid workup, please refer to Chapter 9 in this book.

Q **Question 15.1 OSCE Stem: Examination of a Patient with the following Anterior Segment findings (see Figures 2.16A and 2.16B).**

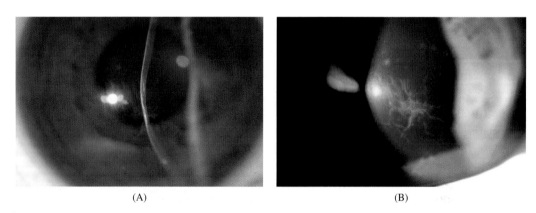

(A)   (B)

Figures 2.16 (A) This patient has keratoconus. The slit beam photograph demonstrates the paracentral thinning with conical apical protrusion and associated stromal scar. (B) The broad beam photograph shows the extent of the scarring with underlying Vogt striae.

On examination of this young patient, there is evidence of **central Vogt striae** with associated **paracentral stromal thinning and apical protrusion with significant corneal scarring**. This is associated with **prominent corneal nerves**. I note a **Fleischer ring at the base of the cone, confirmed under the cobalt blue filter**. Examination of the left eye reveals similar findings. This patient has bilateral keratoconus. I will complete my examination at the slit lamp by flipping the **eyelids to look for papillae** (associated with VKC), performing a dilated fundal examination for associated conditions such as **retinitis pigmentosa, lebers congenital amaurosis (flat ERG)**, and **retinal tears or detachment** associated with chronic eye rubbing. I will check the visual acuity, refraction, relative afferent pupillary defect, associated signs such as oil droplet and scissoring reflex as well as Munson and Rizzutti signs, perform a placido disc examination, take a history of contact lens use, and investigate using a cornea tomography scan.

Q Question 15.2 How would you Manage this Patient with Keratoconus with Significant Stromal Scarring?

Management of keratoconus can be divided into conservative and surgical. For this patient, I will try conservative management with **spectacles, soft toric contact lenses** (likely to fail in view of advanced nature), or **rigid permeable contact lenses depending on the severity of the astigmatism**. If there is progression of the condition, **collagen crosslinking** (central corneal thickness at least **400 μm** thickness as less than 400 μm has increased risk of damaging corneal endothelium, less than 60D keratometry) or insertion of **intrastromal corneal ring segments** (INTACS and KERA ring) can be considered. If the patient is unable to tolerate contact lenses and vision remains poor due to the **stromal scarring or severe astigmatism**, then **optical keratoplasty** can be considered. (Failure of contact lenses is not an indication for collagen crosslinking. Collagen crosslinking indication is mainly to stop progression; 90% of patients can be treated conservatively.)

Q Question 15.3 What are the Surgical Indications for Keratoconus?

Optical keratoplasty is the main surgical treatment for keratoconus. It is indicated in patients who have **severe astigmatism with poor visual acuity despite glasses or contact lenses**, patients who are **unable to tolerate contact lens use**, and patients with **significant stromal scarring involving the visual axis**.

Q Question 15.4 Examine this Patient with a Placido Disc.

Sir, I am going to come close to you with this instrument. Please cover your left eye with your left hand and use your right eye to focus on the lens in the middle and try not to blink. I will come close to you, please do not be afraid. On examination with the placido disc, there are **asymmetric mires with inferonasal steepening**.

I will perform a corneal topography for the patient to look for asymmetric bow tie, thin central cornea, and increased anterior and posterior float. Other investigations will include autorefraction, autokeratometry, placido disc, and corneal pachymetry.

Q **Question 15.6** **How would you Manage Hydrops?**

Management can be divided into acute and chronic management. Acutely I will start the patient on **hypertonic saline**, **broad spectrum preservative-free antibiotics**, **cycoplegics** in the absence of contraindications, and **topical preservative-free steroids**, as well as place a **bandage contact lens**. Chronically, if the scarring is mild, I will attempt to improve vision with glasses or rigid gas-permeable lens. If there is **significant scarring involving the visual axis, poor vision despite contact lenses,** or **intolerance to contact lenses,** I will consider **optical keratoplasty** (do not say lamellar outright as technically hydrops has a break in descemet membrane and hence posterior lamellar is breached as well).

Q. **Question 15.7** **Describe the Orbscan Image in Figure 2.17.**

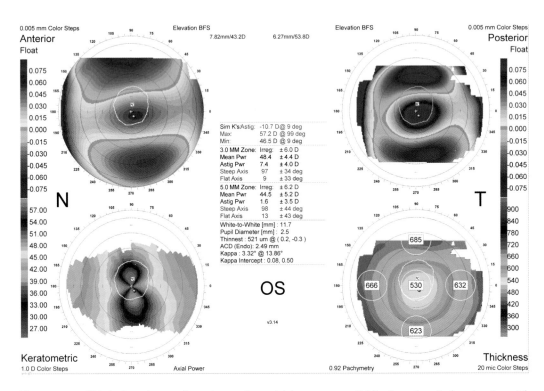

Figure 2.17 This is the orbscan of another patient with keratoconus. While there is apical protrusion with inferior steepening, there is minimal corneal thinning in this case.

This is the orbscan of the left eye showing elevation of both the **anterior and posterior float** above the **best fit sphere**, worse in the posterior float. In the keratometric map, there is presence of **inferior steepening with an asymmetric bowtie appearance**. The pachymetry map shows mild paracentral thinning with the thinnest area measuring 521 μm, corresponding to the protrusion noted on the anterior and posterior float. The Sim K astigmatism is high at −10.7D at axis 9 degrees. Astigmatic measurements in both the 3-mm and 5-mm zones are raised as well. These findings are characteristic of keratoconus.

Q Question 16.1 Viva Stem: What are the Clinical Features of Limbal Stem Cell Deficiency?

The features include loss of palisades of Vogt, whorled epitheliopathy, recurrent or persistent epithelial defect, vascularization, pannus (vascularization and scarring), keratinization, conjunctivalization, corneal melt, and impression cytology showing presence of goblet cells (in chronological and severity order).

Q Question 16.2 How would you Manage a Patient with Limbal Stem Cell Deficiency?

Limbal stem cell deficiency is a difficult condition to manage. Management depends on the underlying cause, visual potential, and symptoms. I will treat the underlying cause. Causes can be divided into congenital and acquired causes. Congenital causes include ectodermal dysplasia, Riley Day syndrome, and aniridia. Acquired causes can be further divided into infective, iatrogenic, and inflammatory causes, and neoplasia (tumors). Infective causes include chlamydia, iatrogenic causes include postsurgical (egkeratoplasty) contact lens wear or long-term topical medications, trauma, chemical injury, and radiation. Inflammatory causes include Steven Johnson syndrome, vernal keratoconjunctivitis, and ocular pemphigoid rosacea.

Management can be divided into conservative and surgical management. If visual acuity is poor and the patient is asymptomatic, I will monitor and treat conservatively with lubricants. If the patient is symptomatic despite conservative treatment, I will treat with **amniotic membrane transplant, Gundersen flap, botulinum injection,** or **lateral tarsorrhaphy,** and **finally evisceration/enucleation**. If the visual potential is good and the patient is asymptomatic, I will treat conservatively with lubricants. If the patient is symptomatic with persistent or recurrent epithelial defects, I will place **a bandage contact lens with topical preservative-free antibiotic cover, and start the patient on oral doxycycline (in the absence of contraindications) and vitamin C, failing which I will consider botulinum injection, temporary tarsorrhaphy,** or **temporary amniotic membrane transplant,** as well as **limbal stem cell transplant**. (Remember to state the treatment measures for the underlying cause if the cause is known.)

I will perform a Gundersen flap operation under informed consent and regional anesthesia in sterile conditions in the operating theater. I will first place a **superior corneal traction suture 7/0 vicryl, debride the corneal surface clean of necrotic tissue or epithelium**, perform a **360 degrees limbal peritomy**, mobilise the **superior conjunctiva, making an incision 14–17 mm above the superior limbus, 2 cm in diameter** (or use 2 mm larger then cornea surface for both height and width; oversize flap as there will be conjunctival contraction postop). Dissecting cleanly, I will separate the conjunctiva from the Tenon's capsule with the aid of subconjunctival lignocaine injection (separate the plane), pulling the flap down over the cornea, and securing with **8/0 vicryl interrupted sutures superiorly to the superior limbus and inferiorly to the inferior conjunctiva**. I will start the patient on **topical antibiotics** and **steroids**. If there is excessive tension, superior relaxing incisions will be required.

Failure may be due to:

1) contraction (secondary to undersizing or cyst formation)
2) inability to remove the corneal epithelium, leading to cyst formation

Q Question 17.1 OSCE Stem: Examination of Young Lady with the following findings (see Figure 2.18); Contralateral Eye Appears Normal.

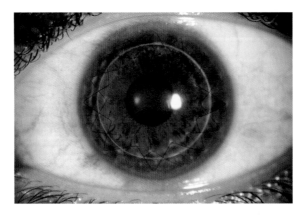

Figure 2.18 This patient had contact lens-related infective keratitis previously that involved the visual axis. She underwent right deep anterior lamellar keratoplasty and the graft remains clear and healthy. Her left eye is normal

On examination of the anterior segment, there is presence of a corneal graft with double running sutures. The sutures are intact and there are no exposed sutures or infiltrates. When a slit is cast at the graft host junction, there is an interface suggestive of a deep anterior lamellar keratoplasty. Otherwise the cornea is clear and there are no keratitic precipitates or signs of rejection. The anterior chamber is deep and quiet. There is no defect noted on transillumination and no glaucoma filtration surgery or aqueous drainage device superiorly. Lids are normal with no aberrant lashes. Examination of the other eye reveals it to be normal. I will complete my examination by checking the intraocular pressure and checking the fundus for increased cup-disc ratio (for steroid-induced glaucoma). In summary, this patient has a left deep anterior lamellar keratoplasty. She is likely to have had a previous stromal scar from causes such as trauma or infective keratitis, or interstitial keratitis or unilateral KC which required a lamellar transplant.

Q Question 17.2 What are the Possible Causes of Infection in the Patient in Question 17.1?

Causes of infective keratitis in the patient can be divided into contact lens-related and non-contact lens-related causes. **Contact lens-related causes are usually bacterial, but can also be fungal or Acanthamoeba** in origin. **Causes of infective keratitis in a non-contact lens user is likely to be viral in nature, such as Herpes simplex.**

	PK	DALK
Sizing of Graft	Oversize	Same Size
Reason	• More endothelial cells in reserve • Increases convexity of button to prevent PAS (smaller graft will result in flatter cornea) • Tighter wound seal for graft	• To avoid a ridge at host graft junction, of which the regenerating epithelial cells are unable to climb across and hence resulting in persistent epithelial defect

Interrupted Sutures	Continuous Sutures
• Technically easier for beginner • For inflamed eyes or eyes with vascularization or pediatric grafts	• Faster and less astigmatism (due to even distribution of tension) • Not for cases where selected suture needs to be removed e.g. infection

Q Question 18.1 Viva Stem: How would you Manage a 70-year-old Patient Presenting with Pain and Loss of Vision (see Figure 2.19)?

This anterior segment photograph shows severe infective keratitis with a superior abscess and opacification of the entire cornea. There is significant thinning of the cornea superiorly

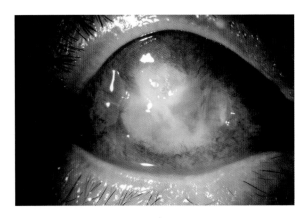

Figure 2.19 This eye has severe infective keratitis with significant amount of thinning which is at risk of perforation. There is neurotrophic keratitis with ulceration.

and nasally. I will examine the eye under the slit lamp, looking at the extent of the thinning, assessing for Seidel sign and the anterior chamber depth, activity, and hypopyon. The eye is chemotic and injected as well. The lids and lashes appear normal otherwise. This patient has severe infective keratitis with impending perforation. I will examine the visual acuity and relative afferent pupillary defect by the reverse method, check the **corneal sensation**, and assess the lids for **lagophthalmos** and **poor Bell's reflex**. I will perform **a gentle B scan** for the right eye. Corneal ulceration is an ocular emergency. I will examine the patient's history for duration of eye symptoms, blurring of vision, previous trauma, history of facial nerve palsy (exposure) or thyroid eye disease, any previous ocular infections and surgeries, or long-term use of eye drops (especially steroids). If the wound is stable and anterior chamber is formed, I will perform **careful scraping** of the ulcer and send for microscopy and cultures. If not, I will swap the area instead. The principles of management are to **treat the infection and underlying predisposing factor, watch for progressive thinning, treat long-term complications**, and **monitor visual rehabilitation depending on visual prognosis.**

> **Q** **Question 18.2 How would you Manage this Patient in whom there is no Lagophthalmos but the Corneal Sensation is Poor?**

This patient has **neurotrophic corneal keratopathy**. Management can be divided into systemic and ocular management. Systemically, I will co-manage with an internist to treat **systemic causes of neurotrophic keratopathy**. I will start the patient on topical preservative-free topical antibiotics (e.g. cravit and cefazolin) and systemic antibiotics. If there is poor response to treatment or progressive thinning, the patient will require a **tectonic** and **therapeutic corneal transplant**, or in the worse case scenario, evisceration.

Q Question 19 OSCE Stem: Examination of Patient (see Figure 2.20).

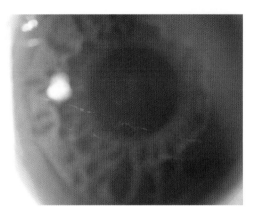

Figure 2.20 Posterior polymorphous corneal dystrophy.

Note: Differential to consider in a patient with more florid features of posterior polymorphous corneal dystrophy: iridocorneal endothelial syndrome.

On examination of the patient's right eye, there is a **thick band-like lesion with thickened edges** in the **posterior stroma extending across the inferior paracentral region**. Otherwise the cornea is clear and there are no other vesicular lesions. The anterior chamber is deep and there is no peripheral anterior synaechiae and no iris atrophy. Patient is phakic with a nuclear sclerotic cataract. There are no iris transillumination defects and no glaucoma filtrating surgery or glaucoma drainage device. Examination of the contralateral eye shows it to be normal. This patient has **posterior polymorphous corneal dystrophy**. I will check the visual acuity and relative afferent pupillary defect, use gonioscopy to look for angle closure, check the intraocular pressure, and perform a dilated fundal examination for increased cup-disc ratio. I will examine the patient's family members and check systemically for **Alport syndrome** (posterior polymorphous corneal dystrophy associated with angle closure glaucoma, AD inheritance, frequently asymmetric, associated with Alport syndrome and fleck retinopathy).

Q Question 20 OSCE stem: Examination of a Patient (see Figures 2.21A and 2.21B).

On examination of the patient's left eye, there is presence of thinning about 50% depth inferiorly extending from 3 to 8 o'clock with **bridging vessels and anterior lipid keratopathy** with **sloping edges** and **no overhanging edges**. Epithelium remains **intact**.

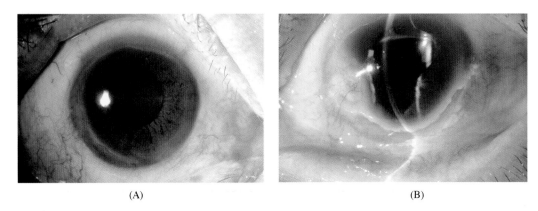

(A)	(B)

Figures 2.21A and 2.21B Bilateral Terrien's marginal degeneration. The condition is usually asymmetrical as seen in this patient where the left eye has more extensive thinning compared to the right eye.

Otherwise **the eye is white, cornea is clear, anterior chamber is deep** and **quiet, and there are no keratic precipitates.** The patient is phakic with a nuclear sclerotic cataract. Examination of the fellow eye reveals similar but asymmetrical findings. The patient has **Terrien's marginal degeneration**. Differentials include peripheral ulcerative keratitis. I will check the visual acuity, refractive error, and intraocular pressure, and perform a dilated fundal examination for vitritis vasculitis and retinitis.

> **Q** **Question 21.1 Viva Stem: Patient with Recurrent Eye Pain and Blurring of Vision that has Worsened over the past few weeks (see Figure 2.22).**

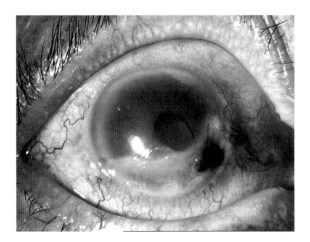

Figure 2.22 Mooren's ulcer is a common cause of peripheral ulcerative keratitis in an Asian population. In this patient, the ulceration has led to focal perforation with prolapse of the uveal tissue. Note the absence of scleritis in this photograph.

This is the anterior segment photograph of the right eye showing an area **of peripheral ulcerative keratitis** extending from 3 to 8 o'clock with an area of **perforation/descematocele** and **iris plugging** at 4 o'clock. It is associated with **overhanging edges** and injected conjunctiva **but no infiltrates, ground glass haze**, or **hypopyon**. The anterior chamber appears shallow with corectopia toward the area of perforation/descematocele. **Lids appear normal** apart from mild meibomian gland disease. I will check the visual acuity, relative afferent papillary defect by the reverse method, **corneal sensation, lid closure**, and **Seidel sign**; examine the anterior chamber for activity; conduct a dilated fundal examination for signs of inflammation and infection; and check the fellow eye. I will **examine the patient systemically** for features of inflammatory conditions such as Wegner's and rheumatoid arthritis. This patient has peripheral ulcerative keratitis with perforation/impending perforation.

Q Question 21.2 How will you Treat this Patient?

I will shield the eye, and start the patient on topical broad-spectrum antibiotics in the absence of contraindications if Seidel test is negative. If it is positive, I will start the patient on oral antibiotics. The patient will need surgical intervention. If the visual prognosis is poor, options include **corneal glue** (if defect is < 2mm), **amniotic membrane transplant**, or **Gundersen flap** (if epithelialised and visual prognosis is poor, it can be left alone). If visual prognosis is good, options include **multilayer amniotic membrane transplant** with anterior chamber reformation, or **lamellar patch graft** or **full thickness tectonic penetrating keratoplasty** for large perforations.

Q Question 21.3 How do you Manage a Patient with Mooren's Ulcer?

Mooren's ulcerative keratitis is a **sight-threatening condition**. It is **difficult to treat** and **requires a stepwise management**. I will need to treat the **inflammation** as well as any **secondary infections**. If there is secondary infection, I will scrape the infiltrate carefully away from sites of thinning or perform conjunctival swabs (safer option) and start the patient on intensive topical antibiotics in the absence of contraindications. For the inflammation, I will refer to the corneal specialist and start the patient on **topical steroids** and **copious amounts of preservative-free lubricants with antibiotic cover** once the infection is under control, failing which I will start **systemic steroids** and **immunosuppressants (caution: steroids can also exacerbate corneal melts/keratolysis)**. If that fails, then excision of adjacent conjunctiva will be required. If there is impending perforation, the patient will require surgical intervention such as glue with bandage contact lens, lamellar patch graft (banana or DALK graft), or full thickness tectonic penetrating keratoplasty.

Management: infection, inflammation/primary cause, thinning, complications (IOP cataracts, etc.).

| | Ocular | |
Systemic	Infective	Non-infective
RA	Bacterial	Rosaecae
SLE	Viruses	Mooren
PAN	Fungal	Terrien
Wegners		MK
RP		+Neurotrophic
Sarcoidosis		+Exposure

Q Question 21.4 How would you Investigate this Patient?

I will perform investigations to look for infection, the underlying cause, and fitness for systemic steroid therapy. I will swab the area of perforation and send off for gram stain and cultures. I will check FBC, ESR, CRP, RF, anti-dsDNA, ANA, pANCA, cANCA, VDRL, LIA IgG IgM, mantoux, chest X-ray and T spot/TB quantiferon to look for the underlying cause. Pre-steroid workup includes FBC, UECr, ESR, CRP, LFT, HIV, syphilis and TB tests as stated earlier, as well as HCV, HBV, UFEME urine c/s, blood pressure, ECG, and blood capillary glucose.

Q Question 22 OSCE Examination: Examination of the Anterior Segment of a Patient with the following findings (see Figures 2.23A and 2.23B).

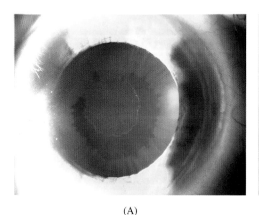

(A)

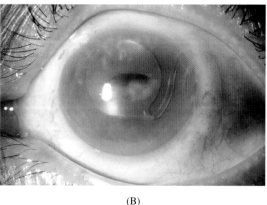

(B)

Figure 2.23 (A) The photo shows the classical Hoarfrost ring seen in eyes with pseudoexfoliation. Pseudoexfoliation presents several challenges to a cataract surgeon — zonulysis, poorly dilating pupil, and glaucoma. This patient has bilateral pseudoexfoliation and had a complicated cataract surgery in the left eye necessitating the implantation of an anterior chamber intraocular lens. (B) The cornea has decompensated and a bandage contact lens was placed to control the pain.

On examination of the patient's right eye, there is presence of **Hoarfrost ring with fibrillary material deposited along the pupillary margin** suggestive of **pseudoexfoliation**. The patient is phakic with a nuclear sclerotic cataract with **no phacodonesis** or **decentration**. The pupil is **well dilated**. There are no iris transillumination defects, glaucoma fitration surgery, or glaucoma drainage device implantation. On examination of the left eye, the cornea is diffusely **edematous** with a bandage contact lens in situ and a central stromal scar with an **angle supported anterior chamber intraocular lens** that is decentered superiorly with a superior nasal **surgical iridectomy** and **absence of posterior capsule**. The anterior chamber is **quiet with no vitreous**. This patient had a complicated left cataract operation requiring an anterior chamber intraocular lens implantation, possibly secondary to left pseudoexfoliation. I will check the visual acuity and relative afferent pupillary defect, perform **gonioscopy for the right eye** for **Sampolesi line** as well as **inferior patchy hyperpigmentation of the trabecular meshwork**, and perform a dilated fundal examination for increased cup-disc ratio as well as formal visual field assessment.

> **Q** **Question 23.1 Viva Stem: Patient with previous Corneal Transplant Presents with Increasing Redness and Pain with Blurring of Vision over the past few days (see Figure 2.24).**

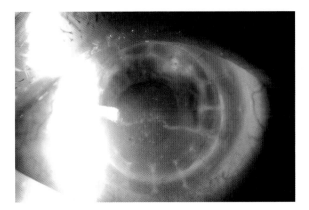

Figure 2.24 This sclerotic scatter image highlights the linear Khodadoust rejection line in a penetrating keratoplasty. This is a sight-threatening condition that can lead to eventual graft failure if left untreated. Note that the line does not extend beyond the graft host junction.

This is the anterior segment photograph of the patient's right eye under sclerotic scatter illumination showing the presence of a corneal graft with **interrupted sutures**, some of which have been removed. There is presence of a **Khodadoust endothelial rejection line** across the visual axis with surrounding medium-sized **keratic precipitates** but it **does not** extend beyond the graft host junction. The graft appears **hazy and edematous. Lids appear normal** and there are **no obvious infiltrates**. I will check the visual acuity, relative afferent pupillary defect, and intraocular pressure; examine under the slit lamp to look for stromal vascularisation and peripheral anterior synechiae, casting a slit to determine the depth of the graft; perform a dilated fundal examination, and check the fellow eye to look for a **likely cause requiring a corneal graft**. In summary, this patient has a **corneal graft with endothelial rejection**.

Q Question 23.2 What are the Risk Factors for Rejection and how would you Manage these?

The risk factors for rejection can be divided into **patient factors** and **ocular factors**. Patient factors include **young patient, patients with multiple grafts,** and **HLA incompatibility**. Ocular factors include **large eccentric grafts, peripheral anterior synechiae, stromal vascularisation, exposed sutures, uncontrolled inflammation,** and **HSV reactivation**.

Endothelial graft rejection is a **sight-threatening condition**. The mainstay of treatment includes **intensive topical steroid with antibiotic cover with or without systemic steroids**. I will admit the patient, start the patient on **hourly Pred Forte eye drops** with antibiotic cover, **perform pre-steroid workup,** and monitor daily for improvement. If there is no improvement, I will consider starting the patient on **systemic oral/intravenous steroid therapy**.

Keratic Precipitates in the Presence of a Corneal Graft	
Rejection	Viral Infection
Classically in a straight line (Khodadoust), IOP not that elevated	CMV endothelitis has more coin-shaped lesions and less stromal keratitis, higher IOP
No dendrites/stromal keratitis	Herpetic endothelitis may have dendrites and stromal keratitis
KPs present on the graft	KPs present on both graft and host cornea

Note: If in doubt, perform an anterior chamber tap for tetraplex and examine the patient's history for previous viral infections.

Q Question 24 OSCE Stem: Examination of a Patient with the Lesion shown in Figure 2.25.

On examination of this patient's left eye, there is presence of a **raised well-defined yellowish white mass lesion with hair follicles** in the **inferotemporal** region straddling the limbus, involving both the cornea and the sclera with an **anterior line of lipid keratopathy**. This features are suggestive of a **limbal dermoid**. Lids appear normal with no **coloboma or**

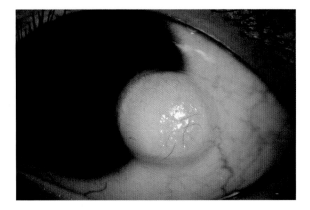

Figure 2.25 Limbal dermoid with an anterior lipid line.

ptosis. I will check the visual acuity and refractive state for **increased astigmatism**, check the extraocular movements for **Duane's syndrome** (associated with Goldenhar syndrome) and nystagmus, perform a dilated fundal examination for optic or foveal hypoplasia and chorioretinal colobomas. I will examine systemically for features of **Goldenhar syndrome** such as **pre-auricular skin tags, deafness, cardiac,** and **spinal abnormalities**.

Q **Question 25 OSCE Stem: Examination of Patient with the following findings (see Figures 2.26A and 2.26B).**

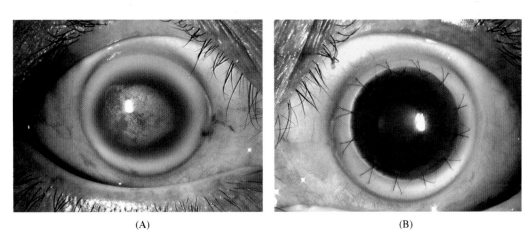

(A)   (B)

Figure 2.26 (A) The right eye has a large central crystalline opacity with associated peripheral lipid deposition. (B) The left eye received a full-thickness corneal graft held by single continuous as well as interrupted sutures.

On examination of the patient's left eye, there is presence of **central corneal crystalline deposits** within the stroma with stromal scarring obscuring the pupil. There is associated **arcus** in the periphery. The epithelium is intact. The anterior chamber is otherwise deep and quiet. On examination of the left eye, there is presence of a corneal graft with a single continuous running suture with interrupted sutures that are intact with peripheral arcus in the host cornea. The graft is clear and well centered with no features of decompensation or rejection. On casting a slit at the junction, it is a full-thickness penetrating keratoplasty. There are no glaucoma drainage device or filtration surgeries in the left eye. This patient is likely to have **Schnyder crystalline corneal dystrophy** status post right penetrating keratoplasty. I will check the visual acuity, perform a dilated fundal examination, and **examine the family members for dyslipidemia**.

> **Q** **Question 26.1 Viva Stem: How would you Manage a Foreign Worker involved in an industrial accident with Chemical Splash Injury (see Figure 2.27)?**

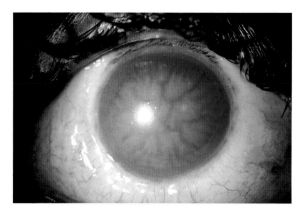

Figure 2.27 Grade 4 chemical injury based on Roper-Hall grading with 360-degrees limbal ischemia and opacified cornea. The anterior chamber is poorly visualized.

This is the anterior segment photograph of the patient's right eye showing diffuse **opacified cornea with total epithelial defect** with associated **360 degrees of limbal ischemia**. Otherwise the lids and lashes appear grossly normal. There is a **poor view of the anterior chamber**. I will check systemically for **life-threatening injuries** and **lid injuries**, assess the visual acuity and relative afferent pupillary defect by the reverse method, check the intraocular pressure, carry out **staining with fluorescein**, perform a **B scan**, and check the fellow eye. This patient has **grade 4 chemical injury** based on **Roper-Hall grading**.

Q Question 26.2 How would you Manage Acutely?

Chemical injury is an **ocular emergency**. **Principles of management include excluding life-threatening injuries, excluding other sight-threatening injuries, removal of offending agent, controlling inflammation, treating concomitant infections, promoting healing, providing substrates for healing, treating long-term complications**, and **visual rehabilitation**. I will take a quick patient's history regarding **duration of injury, any prior irrigation**, and **what the offending agent was** (acid or alkali). Acutely I will start copious **irrigation with at least 1 L of normal saline, everting the lids and sweeping the fornices, till the litmus turns neutral**. I will start the patient on copious amounts of preservative-free **lubricants** with broad-spectrum **antibiotic** cover in the absence of contraindications, preservative-free **steroids**, 1 g vitamin C, and oral doxycycline; admit the patient; and review daily with daily roding and removal of pseudomembranes. If there is poor healing of the epithelium, I will consider inserting a bandage contact lens, botulinum injection to the lids and lateral tarrsoharphy.

Note: Can consider inserting symblepharon ring.

Q Question 26.3 What is the Difference between Alkali and Acid?

Alkali results in saponification of the lipid cell membrane and penetrates deeper, resulting in more extensive damage. Acid coagulates cellular proteins, creating a barrier to further penetration.

CHAPTER 3

GLAUCOMA

Q **Question 1.1 Viva Stem: How do you Manage a Patient who presents with Acute Blurring of Vision, Headache, and Halos (see Figure 3.1)?**

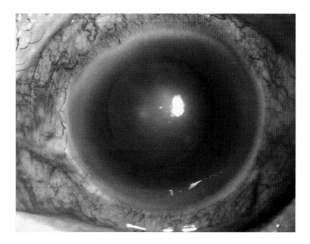

Figure 3.1 This patient has signs typical of acute primary angle closure — injected conjunctiva, mild dilated pupil, and a slightly hazy cornea.

Figure 3.1 shows the anterior segment photograph of the patient's left eye showing an injected eye with hazy cornea and a **mid-dilated pupil** with a nuclear sclerotic cataract. I will check the visual acuity and relative afferent papillary defect by the **reverse method**, cast a slit to assess the **anterior chamber depth** and activity, check for **phacodonesis** and **intraocular pressure**, examine the fundus for **increased cup-disc ratio**, examine the fellow eye (looking for anterior chamber depth), and perform a **gonioscopy**.

Acute angle closure is an **ocular emergency**. The principles of management would be to **decrease the intraocular pressure** to **clear the cornea** for **definitive laser peripheral iridotomy**. In the absence of contraindications, I will administer **intravenous acetazolamide 500 mg stat** and start the patient on **anti-glaucoma eye drops** such as timolol and brimonidine, **pred forte and start pilocarpine 4%** when the intraocular pressure is below 30 mmHg. I will lay the patient supine and perform corneal indentation to reduce the pressure. I will treat the contralateral eye with pilocarpine 2% three times a day. In the meantime, I will check the **renal function, electrocardiogram, and chest X-ray.** I will recheck the pressure after one hour, and if the pressure remains high, I will give a second dose of intravenous acetazolamide with potassium chloride tablet. If the pressure remains high after two doses of acetazolamide, I will administer intravenous **20% mannitol 0.5–2 g/kg over 30 minutes**. When the intraocular pressure has reduced and the cornea is clear, I will perform definitive laser peripheral iridotomy to relieve the pupil block.

Q Question 1.2 If the Pressure does not Drop after Mannitol and Maximum Diamox, What can be Tried?

I will lay the patient supine and perform **indentation of the cornea to promote aqueous outflow**. If the pressure remains elevated, I can perform **anterior chamber paracentesis** to relieve the pressure or laser iridoplasty to open the angles prior to attempting a peripheral laser iridotomy. (If the pressure remains high, pilocarpine will not work to break the attack.)

Principles

- Lower eye pressure
- Relief pupil block
- Protect fellow eye
- Follow up long term to prevent chronic angle closure glaucoma

Q Question 1.3 How would you Perform a Laser Peripheral Iridotomy (LPI) Procedure?

I will perform a **sequential argon-YAG laser peripheral iridotomy** under informed consent. I will **pretreat with brimonidine** in the absence of contraindications and **pilocarpine 2% to the non-attacked eye and 4% to the attacked eye**. I will position the patient comfortably at the **argon laser**, using a **high plus lenticule lens** (Abraham iridotomy lens +66 or Wise lens), under topical anesthesia, choosing a location **superior nasal** or **superior temporal at 1/3 2/3 junction from the limbus in an iris cleft**, using initial settings of **800 mW 50 microns 50 ms**, to create a peripheral iridotomy with the **end point of a plume** and deepening of the anterior chamber. I will then switch over to the YAG machine and enlarge the peripheral iridotomy with settings of **2.4 mJ**. I will monitor the patient and **check the intraocular pressure 30 minutes later** and treat with **topical antibiotics and steroids for two weeks**. I will review the patient in **two–three days with gonioscopy OA**. (Review in two-three days to assess IOP in patients with APAC; review in two weeks for patients with PACS only.)

Q Question 1.4 If Angles are still Closed after LPI.

In our center, if angles remain closed after laser peripheral iridotomy, we will **monitor the patient and consider cataract surgery if there is a visually significant cataract**. However, other options would include a **laser iridoplasty** as well. (Practice may vary between different institutions.)

Q Question 1.5 If View is too Hazy for LPI.

Other options such as **laying the patient supine** and **indenting on the globe to improve aqueous outflow, scraping of the epithelium** to clear the view, or **laser peripheral iridoplasty** can be considered. Failing which, **laser pupilloplasty or anterior chamber paracentesis** can be considered.

Q Question 1.6 How do you Perform AC Paracentesis in a PAC Eye?

I will perform anterior chamber paracentesis under informed consent at the slit lamp under topical anesthesia and sterile conditions. I will use a **27-gauge needle mounted on an insulin syringe with the plunger removed**, and enter at a **peripheral site where the anterior chamber is the deepest, avoiding contact with the iris or lens capsule** with the end point of clearing of the cornea.

Q Question 1.7 How would you Perform LPI Differently in an APAC Eye?

If the cornea is hazy, I will **scrape the epithelium and perform anterior chamber paracentesis if required**. I will choose the area of clearest cornea and deepest anterior chamber with increased power settings to place the iridotomy. I will monitor post-laser to watch for intraocular pressure spike.

Q **Question 1.8 What are the Side Effects of LPI?**

The common side effects of laser peripheral iridotomy include **glare, haloes, and diplopia**. Other complications include **inflammation, transient increased intraocular pressure, and hyphema**. Sight-threatening complications include **foveal burns, aqueous misdirection, bullous keratopathy, and cataract (+/–zonulysis)**.

Q **Question 2.1 OSCE Stem: Examination of the Anterior Segment of the Patient.**

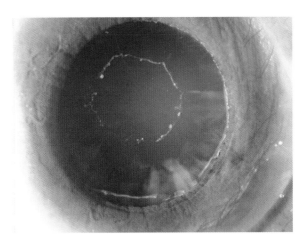

Figure 3.2 This anterior segment image demonstrates features of pseudoexfoliation such as Hoarfrost ring and fibrillary material deposited along the papillary edge. The pupil is mid-dilated as a result, and it could pose a significant challenge during cataract surgeries.

On examination of the anterior segment, this patient has features of pseudoexfoliation as evidenced by presence of a **hoarfrost ring, fibrillary material along the pupil margins, iris sphincter atrophy,** and **pigments on the corneal endothelium**. There is no **trabeculectomy or glaucoma drainage device** present. The **pupil is mid-dilated** with a nuclear sclerotic cataract. There is no obvious **phacodonesis** or **asymmetry of the anterior chamber depth**. Examination of the contralateral eye shows it to be normal. I will check the visual acuity, relative afferent pupillary defect, and intraocular pressure; perform a gonioscopy for **Sampaolesi line, patchy hyperpigmentation of the trabecular meshwork especially inferiorly (versus uniform hyperpigmentation of the trabecular meshwork in pigment dispersion syndrome)**; examine the fundus **for increased cup-disc ratio;** perform a **standard automated perimetry;** and examine systemically for cardiovascular disease **(systemic associations: aortic aneurysm)**.

Note: PDS has phacodonesis (pigments can weaken zonules). Check fundus for myopic changes. Glaucoma secondary to pigment dispersion syndrome: open angle (pigments deposits on the trabecular meshwork), angle closure (subluxed lens).

Q Question 2.2 Management of Pseudoexfoliation with Cataract.

The issues with pseudoexfoliation for cataract surgery are **poorly dilating pupils, zonulysis, increased intraocular pressure, postoperative inflammation, and capsular phimosis**. Management can be divided into preoperative, perioperative, intraoperative, and postoperative stages.

Preoperatively, I will assess the degree of zonular weakness by performing an ultrasound biomicroscopy, access the endothelial cell count, check the anterior chamber intraocular lens biometry, and have on standby an anterior vitrectomy. If the pupils are poorly dilating, I will start topical atropine 1% in the absence of contraindications three days before surgery. I will also control the intraocular pressure with topical glaucoma eye drops.

Perioperatively, I will start the patient on intravenous mannitol 0.5–2 g/kg 20% over 20 min if the intraocular pressure is raised, and instill 10% phenylephrine if the pupils are poorly dilated.

Intraoperatively, I will perform the surgery under informed consent under regional anesthesia in sterile conditions. If the pupil remains small, I will inject 1:10000 adrenaline with balanced salt solution intracamerally. If that fails, I will dilate the pupils by viscodilation, failure of which I will attempt stretching with Kuglen hooks or sphincterotomy. If that fails, I will then insert a Malyugin ring or iris hook.

If there is zonular weakness, management depends on the extent. If it is less than three clock hours, I will perform a careful phacoemulsification. I will initiate the rhexis with a needle, completing it by starting small and gradually enlarging. I will then place capsular hooks to stabilize the bag followed by gentle hydrodissection. I will perform the surgery under reduced settings, using an *in situ* chop technique with a sharp second instrument to reduce zonular stress. After removal of the soft lens material, I will insert a **capsular bag expansion device (CTR) followed by a three-piece intraocular lens**. If there is **three to six clock hours of zonulysis**, I will perform extracapsular cataract extraction, and either leave the patient **aphakic for future secondary fixated intraocular lens implantation** or **insert an anterior chamber intraocular lens**. If there is more than six clock hours of weakness, I will perform intracapsular cataract extraction. Other methods include insertion of Cionni 1 L or 2 L as well.

Postoperatively, I will monitor the patient for prolonged inflammation as well as capsular phimosis or posterior capsular opacification.

> **Q** **Question 3.1** Viva Stem: Patient with a History of Uveitic Glaucoma underwent a Primary Tube Implantation in the Right Eye. He presents two days after his operation complaining of Pain and Blurring of Vision. What are the Possible Differentials?

I would first exclude sight-threatening conditions related to the surgery such as endophthalmitis (though the duration is rather short), raised intraocular pressures secondary to hyphema, suprachoroidal hemorrhage, or aqueous misdirection, as well as reactivation of his underlying uveitic condition or surgically induced necrotizing scleritis. Other common causes include corneal abrasions as well as traumatic iritis.

> **Q** **Question 3.2** Examination of the Patient reveals findings shown in Figure 3.3 with IOP of 45 mmHg.

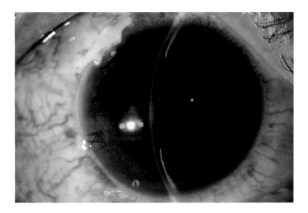

Figure 3.3 This patient developed aqueous misdirection after a tube implantation. Note the grade 2 uniformly shallow anterior chamber that is typical of malignant glaucoma.

This is the anterior segment photograph of the patient's eye showing a **grade 2 flat anterior chamber with pupillo-corneal touch** with a slightly hazy cornea and injected conjunctiva. There is a superior temporal tube seen that appears patent with good conjunctival coverage. In view of the raised intraocular pressure, this is likely an **aqueous misdirection**. I will check the visual acuity and relative afferent papillary defect, and examine the fundus **to exclude suprachoroidal hemorrhage**. I will perform an ultrasound biomicroscopy to look for anterior rotation of the ciliary body and loss of the ciliary sulcus.

Q **Question 3.3 How would you Treat?**

Aqueous misdirection is an ocular emergency. Management can be divided into medical and surgical management. I will first start the patient on **topical glaucoma medications** in the absence of contraindications together with **topical atropine to rotate the ciliary body back**. I will administer **intravenous acetazolamide** 500 mg, failing which I can give a second dose after one hour before giving intravenous mannitol 20% 0.5–2 g/kg over 20–30 mins. If these fail, I can try to **enlarge the peripheral iridotomy/iridectomy**. (If the patient is **pseudokphakic, I will perform a YAG capsulotomy and anterior hyloidotomy**. However, do not mention in this case as THIS patient is phakic). Failing which I will refer the patient to the retinal surgeon for an urgent **pars plana vitrectomy**.

Note: Another option rarely used nowadays is Chandler's procedure.

Q **Question 3.4 What is Malignant Glaucoma?**

Aqueous misdirection is a serious but rare complication of ocular surgeries. It occurs secondary to **anterior rotation of the ciliary body** with ciliolenticular obstruction resulting in posterior diversion of the aqueous into the anterior hyaloid face, and also resulting in **anterior shift of the lens iris diaphragm with resultant angle closure in the presence of a patent iridotomy/iridectomy**.

> Risk factors for aqueous misdirection:
>
> Intact anterior hyloid with vitreous syneresis, previous aqueous misdirection in fellow eye, small crowded eye (nanophthalmic), long redundant posteriorly directed ciliary processes

Q **Question 3.5 What are the Risk Factors for Aqueous Misdirection in Patients Going for Surgery?**

Patients at risk are patients with a **shallow anterior chamber, nanophthalmic eyes (small normal eyes), previous history of aqueous misdirection, anterior vitreous face,** and **long posteriorly oriented ciliary process**.

Q **Question 4 OSCE Stem: Examination of Patient with Hypertension and Diabetes presenting with Blurring of Vision (see Figure 3.4).**

This is the anterior segment photograph of the patient's right eye showing the presence of extensive rubeosis iridis with associated ectropion uvea and posterior synechia at 7 o' clock. The cornea is clear with no evidence of decompensation from raised intraocular pressure.

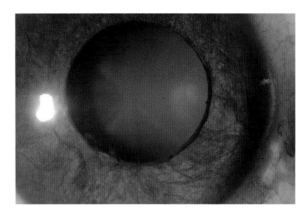

Figure 3.4 Neovascular glaucoma secondary to central retinal vein occlusion.

The anterior chamber is shallow but quiet and the patient has a mild nuclear sclerotic cataract. There is no evidence of glaucoma filtration surgery or drainage device implantation. I will check the visual acuity, relative afferent papillary defect, and intraocular pressure, conduct a gonioscopy and dilated fundal examination looking for a cause (e.g. DR, OIS, old CRVO), and check the fellow eye, auscultating for carotid bruit and performing an automated perimetry.

Management of neovascular glaucoma is **difficult** and carries a **poor prognosis**. Management depends on the underlying cause, the visual prognosis, and ocular symptoms. **Common causes** include **ocular ischemic syndrome, proliferative diabetic retinopathy**, and **central retinal vein occlusion**. Other causes include chronic RD, uveitis, eales, radiation, and tumors. Management can be divided into **systemic** and **ocular management**. I will co-manage with a physician to control the patient's systemic vascular risk factors. I will also perform **urgent pan-retinal photocoagulation**. If the visual prognosis is poor with no ocular symptoms, I will treat conservatively with ocular pressure-lowering medications and monitor for bullous keratopathy and secondary infections. If the patient is symptomatic, I will consider **transscleral cyclophotocoagulation**, failing which I will consider a Gundersen flap (retrobulbar alcohol injection or evisceration/enucleation is much rarer). If the visual prognosis is good, I will treat with ocular pressure-lowering drops, failing which I will consider high-risk **glaucoma filtration surgery with mitomycin C** or implantation of a **glaucoma drainage device**. I will refer the patient to a vitreoretinal surgeon to consider treatment with **intravitreal antivascular endothelial growth factor**.

> **Q** **Question 5.1 Viva Stem: How do you Manage a Patient presenting with Acute Blurring of Vision and Pain (see Figure 3.5)?**

This is the anterior segment photograph of the patient's left eye showing a mid-dilated pupil, shallow anterior chamber, **more shallow inferiorly than superiorly,** diffusely hazy edematous cornea, dense nuclear sclerotic cataract, and injected conjunctiva. I will check

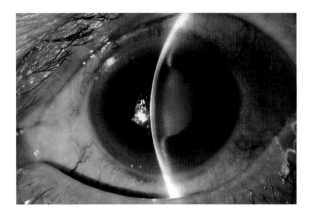

Figure 3.5 This patient has acute secondary angle closure secondary to a dense subluxed lens. The other eye is normal with a deep anterior chamber.

the visual acuity, relative afferent papillary defect by the reverse method, and intraocular pressure, perform a gonioscopy, check the anterior segment for **features of pseudoexfoliation** (causes for the dislocation) and signs of trauma, examine the fundus for cup-disc ratio and signs of trauma (e.g. retinal tear/detachment), perform a B scan if there is no view, examine the fellow eye for possible etiologies, and lay the patient down to assess for anterior–posterior displacement.

This patient has a left **subluxed phakic lens with secondary angle closure and raised intraocular pressure**. This is an **ocular emergency** and principles of management will be to **lower the intraocular pressure urgently** and **clear the cornea for subsequent definitive cataract surgery**. I will examine the patient's history for the duration of symptoms as well as presence of any previous ocular surgeries, trauma, or disease. Acutely I will lower the **intraocular pressure with topical anti-glaucoma medications and intravenous acetazolamide with topical steroids** in the absence of contraindications. I will lay the patient supine. If this fails, I will administer intravenous mannitol. Once the cornea is clear, I will perform an **endothelial cell count** and **ultrasound biomicroscopy to assess the degree of zonulysis, obtain biometry for anterior chamber intraocular lens**, and **have on standby an anterior vitrectomy**. Perioperatively, I will start the patient on **intravenous mannitol**. Intraoperative management will depend on the number of clock hours of zonulysis. If zonulysis is less than three clock hours, I will perform careful phacoemulsification with insertion of capsular bag expansion device. If zonulysis is between three and six clock hours, I will perform an extracapsular cataract extraction. If zonulysis is more than six clock hours, I will perform an intracapsular cataract extraction. Other methods would include insertion of a Cionni 1 L or 2 L capsular tension ring (need for anchorage points to sclera). Postoperatively, I will monitor the intraocular pressure and centration of the lens, and look for complications such as retinal detachment and cystoids macula edema (as well as suture complications in sclera/iris fixed IOLs).

I will perform **careful phacoemulsification** for this patient in the operating theater under informed consent using regional anesthesia in sterile conditions. If the view is still hazy, I will **scrape the epithelium**, using **vision blue to stain the capsule** if visualization is poor. I will initiate my rhexis using a needle, **starting small and gradually enlarging**. After that, I will insert **capsular hooks to stabilize the capsular bag**, perform a good hydrodissection, insert a **capsular bag expansion device to open up the bag** followed by subsequent phacoemulsification using *in situ* **chop technique** with a sharp second instrument with lowered parameters to reduce zonular stress and avoiding excessive downward pressure. I will **insert a three-piece intraocular lens** followed by aspiration of viscoelastic, ensuring complete removal to avoid postoperative pressure spike. (If performing ECCE or ICCE, I can opt for ACIOL or leave aphakic for future secondary fixated IOL implantation.)

Q Question 6 Viva Stem: How would you Manage a Patient presenting with Increasing Pain with Blurring of Vision (see Figure 3.6)?

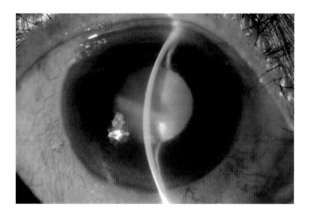

Figure 3.6 This is the typical presentation of phacomorphic glaucoma. Note the presence of uniformly shallow anterior chamber, and hazy edematous cornea with a white intumescent lens.

This patient has **right phacomorphic glaucoma**. This is an **ocular emergency** and requires **urgent reduction of intraocular pressure to clear the cornea for subsequent definite cataract surgery**. I will first take the patient's history of duration of symptoms and trauma. I will examine the visual acuity, assessing for perception of light in all four quadrants, check the relative afferent pupillary defect by the reverse method, perform a gonioscopy, check for phacodonesis, and compare with the contralateral eye as well as perform a **B scan to assess the retinal status**. In the absence of contraindications, I will lay the patient **supine** and start the patient on **topical glaucoma medications and steroids, and intravenous acetazolamide,** failing which I will administer intravenous 20% mannitol (0.5–2 g/kg).

Once the intraocular pressure is controlled and cornea is clear, I will arrange for early cataract operation. Factors to consider can be divided into preoperative, perioperative, intraoperative, and postoperative stages.

Preoperatively, I will assess the **endothelial cell count and degree of zonular weakness using ultrasound biomicroscopy, check the biometry for anterior chamber intraocular lens, and order an anterior vitrectomy on standby.** Perioperatively, I will start the patient on **intravenous mannitol.** Intraoperatively, I will perform the surgery under informed consent and regional anesthesia in sterile conditions. I will **scrape the epithelium** if the view is hazy secondary to corneal edema, create a **long corneal tunnel, and place it anteriorly** (to prevent iris prolapse and prevent hitting the iris or anterior capsule). I will **stain the capsule with vision blue,** fill the anterior chamber with cohesive viscoelastic to maintain the chamber and dispersive viscoelastic to coat the endothelium. I will first decompress the capsule with **a 27-gauge needle mounted on a 3-mL syringe,** then perform the capsulorrhexis, starting small and gradually enlarging. I will avoid hydrodissection (as the cortex is liquefied and there might be a posterior polar cataract) for this patient and complete the surgery by performing a careful phacoemulsification. Intraoperatively, I will refill viscoelastic frequently and avoid excessive pressure fluctuations. At the end of surgery, I will ensure complete removal of viscoelastic and good intraocular pressure. Postoperatively, I will monitor for glaucoma and corneal decompensation and prolonged inflammation.

Q Question 7.1 Viva Stem: What is Transscleral Cyclophotocoagulation? What are other Newer Types of Modalities?

Transscleral cyclophotocoagulation is a **cyclodestructive procedure** using a **fiber optic G probe diode laser.** Newer modalities include endoscopic, micropulse, or ultrasound.

Q Question 7.2 How would you Perform Transscleral Cyclophotocoagulation?

I will perform transscleral cyclophotocoagulation under informed consent in the operating theater under topical anesthesia in sterile conditions. Using a **fiber optic G probe diode laser with transillumination** to identify the ciliary body, at a distance **1.5 mm posterior to the limbus,** using a setting of **1500–2000 mW, 1500–2000 ms,** aiming to apply **10 shots per quadrant,** treating 270–360 degrees while **avoiding 3 and 9 o' clock position,** aiming to hear a **pop sound 50% of the time** representing **microablation of the ciliary body epithelium.** I will then cover the patient with analgesia, cycloplegics, tobradex 4 times a day, **continue all glaucoma eyedrops** and review him the next day. (Transillumination to mark junction of black and white ie ciliary body. Especially for conditions such as trauma, anterior segment dysgenesis, congenital glaucoma and neovascular glaucoma where there might be anatomical distortion.)

Q Question 7.3 When is Transscleral Cyclophotocoagulation Indicated?

Transscleral cyclophotocoagulation is traditionally indicated for patients with a **painful blind eye secondary to uncontrolled raised intraocular pressure**.

Q Question 7.4 When is Transscleral Cyclophotocoagulation Contraindicated?

Transcleral cyclophotocoagulation is contraindicated in patients with uveitis due to risk of hypotony (ciliary body shutdown) and phthisis bulbi as well as in patients with thin sclera or silicone oil (risk of scleral melt).

Q Question 7.5 What are the Complications of Transscleral Cyclophotocoagulation?

The most serious complication is hypotony with subsequent phthisis development as well as sympathetic ophthalmia. Common complications include pain. Other complications include iritis, vitritis, cystoid macular edema, and scleral melt, as well as conjunctival burns, hyphema, and malignant glaucoma.

Q Question 8.1 Viva Stem: What are the Types of Gonioscopy Lenses?

Gonioscopy lenses can be divided into **direct and indirect** lenses. Direct lenses include **Koppe as well as therapeutic lenses like Barkan lens**. Indirect lenses can be divided into indentational and non-indentational. Indentational lenses include Sussman, Posner, and Volk 4 mirror lenses. Non-indentational lenses include Volk 2 or 3 mirror lenses.

	Indirect	
Direct	Indentational	Non-indentational
Koppe	Sussman	Goldman/Volk 2 or 3
Barkan	Posner	mirror
	Volk 4 mirror	

Q Question 8.2 How would you Perform Selective Laser Trabeculoplasty (SLT)?

I will perform **selective laser trabeculoplasty** under informed consent under topical anesthesia, pretreat with brimonidine eye drops, using double frequency YAG laser machine, aiming to put in 25 shots per quadrant with a setting of **0.5–1.0 mJ, 400 microns, 3 ns using a Latina lens** aiming at the trabecular meshwork and looking for the **end point of champagne bubble sign**. I will then start the patient on topical steroids and monitor the patient. (SLT effect lasts about two years.)

Q **Question 8.3 How would you Perform Laser Iridoplasty?**

I will perform laser iridoplasty under informed consent and topical anesthesia using the argon laser machine. Using a **high plus lenticule lens (Abraham iridotomy lens),** with a setting of **300–500 mW, 300–500 ms, 300–500 microns** titrating as required, I will **administer 8–12 shots in the periphery**. (The aim is for **photocoagulative effect of laser to cause contraction of the collagen** to pull iris away from the angles.)

Q **Question 9.1 Viva Stem: How would you Perform a Trabeculectomy?**

I will perform trabeculectomy under informed consent in the operating theater under sterile conditions with **peribulbar anesthesia**. I will first place a **superior corneal traction suture with 7/0 vicryl,** create a **superior-nasal fornix-based conjunctival peritomy, create a partial thickness 5 by 3 mm scleral flap first with a beaver blade, then completing the lamellar dissection at 2/3 1/3 depth with a crescent blade up till the limbus**. I will then place sponges soaked with **mitomycin C 0.4 mg/mL** under the conjunctival and scleral flap **for two minutes, taking care to avoid the conjunctival edge and cornea**. I will then **irrigate with at least 50 mL of balanced salt solution and create an anterior chamber paracetensis at a distal site to decompress the eye** (to prevent suprachoroidal as entering will create a sudden drop in IOP) before **entering the anterior chamber through the scleral flap using a Beaver blade and enlarging the sclerostomy with a Kelly's punch**. I will then create a **surgical iridectomy and suture the scleral flap edges with 10/0 nylon before reforming the anterior chamber through the paracentesis and checking for aqueous egression**. I will then ensure a **water-tight closure of the conjunctiva using mattress and purse string method using 10/0 nylon**. I will then **inject subconjunctival cefazolin and dexamethasone inferiorly and stop all glaucoma medications and review the next day**. (In combined phaco-trab, phaco can be performed before the trab, after sclera flap creation with a separate incision or through the sclerostomy.)

Q **Question 9.2 What is your Management of a Patient Post-Trabeculectomy Presenting with Shallow Anterior Chamber?**

Management of shallow anterior chamber post-trabeculectomy depends on the underlying cause, whether the **pressure is high or low**, and **grade of shallow anterior chamber**. If the pressure is low, causes include **overfiltration** (high bleb no leak) **or bleb leak (low bleb) or under secretion** (ciliary body shutdown or cyclodialysis cleft) or retinal detachment (hypotony). If the pressure is high, the causes include **suprachoroidal haemorrhage** and **pupil block** (hyphema, fibrin, iris can block PI) as well as **aqueous misdirection**. I will check the visual acuity and relative afferent pupillary defect, examine the **bleb height** and assess if it is high or low, **paint the bleb looking for Seidel sign**, examine the anterior chamber for **uniformly shallow anterior chamber, fibrin, and hyphema, check the patency of the iridectomy, check the intraocular pressure**, and **perform a dilated fundal examination for choroidal detachments**.

Note: State low pressure causes first as they are the most common.

Q   **Question 9.3   Based on Figure 3.7, How will you Manage?**

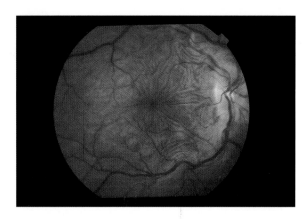

Figure 3.7   Fundal photo of the eye with hypotonous maculopathy.

This is the fundal photograph of the right eye showing subretinal **linear striae suggestive of choroidal folds** involving the fovea with **vessel tortuosity** and **disc edema**. I will examine under the slit lamp with a 78 dioptre lens looking for **cystoid macula edema** and examining the periphery for **choroidal detachment**. I will check for **bleb height and paint the bleb looking for positive Seidel test**. This patient has hypotonous maculopathy.

Management can be divided into medical and surgical management, and is dependent on the underlying cause and degree of anterior chamber shallowing.

The photos (**please refer to the next page**) show the right cystic bleb painted with fluorescein stain under cobalt blue light showing Seidel's positive leakage centrally. This patient has hypotony secondary to a bleb leak.

I will first treat conservatively by reducing steroids and increasing antibiotics such as tobramycin/gentamicin and starting the patient on atropine (cycloplegics to deepen AC)

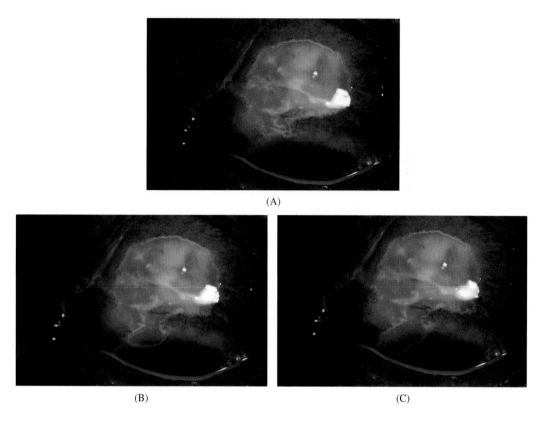

(A)

(B)   (C)

Figures 3.8A–3.8C Three sequential photos illustrating a leak at the mid-temporal edge of a cystic avascular bleb in the right eye — Seidel's positive.

in the absence of contraindications and starting aqueous suppressants (ABCs — alpha2 agonist, beta blockers, CAI). If that fails, I can place a pressure bandage contact lens or a Simmonds shell to reduce the rate of leak. I will treat **surgically if there is grade 3 anterior chamber shallowing with lenticular corneal touch** and **persistent hypotony especially in an only eye patient**. I will consider anterior chamber reformation with viscoelastic air or basic salt solution with resuturing of the bleb/bleb revision (excision and conjunctival advancement for late bleb leakages).

(Separate scenario: If the bleb is overfilled with no leak, the cause is likely overfiltration. I will treat conservatively first by increasing antibiotics and reducing steroids and starting atropine and aqueous suppressants. If that fails, I will apply a pressure pad (torpedo patch) or bolster, failing which I will reform the anterior chamber with viscoelastic or gas or consider injection of **autologous blood**. If the anterior chamber remains shallow, I can then either place mattress compression sutures or resuture the scleral flaps/bleb revision. However, in general, I will consider early surgical intervention in only-eye-ed patients, persistent hypotony with hypotonus maculopathy, grade 3 shallow anterior chamber, profuse leakage especially in fornix-based trabeculectomies.)

Q **Question 9.4** **What are the Complications of Trabeculectomy?**

Complications of trabeculectomy can be divided into intraoperative, and early and late postoperative stages.

Intraoperative complications include **button hole of the conjunctival** or **scleral flap, hyphema, suprachoroidal haemorrhage, retrobulbar haemorrhage, entry of mitomycin C,** and **globe perforation**.

Early postoperative complications include **hypotony secondary to wound leak or overfiltration, raised intraocular pressure secondary to aqueous misdirection, suprachoroidal hemorrhage,** and **pupil block, and under filtration, hyphema, endophthalmitis, retinal detachment,** and **wipeout**. Late postoperative complications include **bleb leak, blebitis, late onset bleb-related endophthalmitis, bleb failure, cataract,** and **progression of glaucoma**.

(The patient had a trabeculectomy many years ago. He now comes in with acute red painful eyes: differentials include blebitis, BRE, corneal abrasion/epitheliopathy, especially if the patient is on multiple glaucoma drops, failed trabeculectomy with raised intraocular pressure, uveitis.)

(Blebitis: look for local risk factors such as lid disease, trichiasis, exposure, cystic overhanging avascular blebs, and bleb leak, as well as use of anti-metabolites. Look for systemic risk factors such as immunocompromised state e.g. DM. Admit the patient, need to exclude BRE, keep in view tap and jab. Patient will require **definitive bleb revision; keep in view graft for possible melted scleral flap**. Topical moxifloxacin is preferred as levofloxacin does not cover gram positive well.)

Note: Complications of tube e.g. corneal decompensation; investigations include ASOCT, corneal pachymetry, and endothelial cell count.

Q **Question 9.5** **When would you Intervene Surgically in a Postoperative Bleb Leakage?**

I will consider early surgical intervention if the **anterior chamber is shallow with lenticular corneal touch (grade 3), if he is an only-eye-ed patient, and if there is persistent hypotony with cystoid macular edema or maculopathy, especially if it is a fornix-based flap with brisk leakage.**

Grading of AC

- Grade 1: iridocorneal touch
- Grade 2: pupillocorneal touch
- Grade 3: lenticulocorneal touch

In this patient, I will be worried about **aqueous misdirection**. I will confirm my diagnosis by performing an **ultrasound biomicroscopy** for **anteriorly rotated ciliary body with loss of the ciliary sulcus**. This is an **ocular emergency**. Treatment can be divided into conservative and surgical. I will start the patient on **maximum topical as well as systemic anti-glaucoma medications in the absence of contraindications as well as topical atropine**. If that fails to control the pressure, if the patient is pseudophakic, I will perform **YAG capsulotomy and anterior hyloidotomy**. If that fails or if the patient is phakic, I will refer to the vitreoretinal surgeon for **pars plana vitrectomy**. (Try not to mention Chandler's unless it is requested.)

Q **Question 11.1** Viva Stem: How will you Manage a 50-year-old Patient presenting Post-Trauma with Pain and Blurring of Vision (see Figure 3.9)?

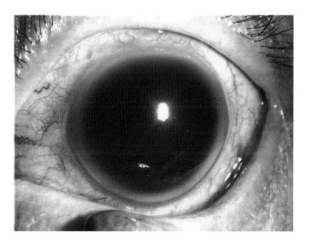

Figure 3.9 This patient has total hyphema after blunt trauma which completely obscures the view of the iris and the anterior chamber.

This is the anterior segment photograph of the patient's left eye showing a hazy cornea with **total hyphema** with **no view of the anterior segment**. There are otherwise no evidence of globe rupture or lid injuries from this photograph and the eye does not appear proptotic. I will exclude life-threatening injuries, look for orbital injuries (e.g. EOM limitation secondary to entrapment), check visual acuity and light projection and relative afferent papillary defect by the reverse method, check intraocular pressure, and perform a B scan to look for retinal tears/detachments and vitreous hemorrhage. I examine the patient's history for **mechanism of injury, duration of injury, progression of symptoms,** and **any prior treatments and any other injuries** and whether the patient is on **anticoagulants**.

Q Question 11.2 How would you Manage an Intraocular Pressure of 35?

Traumatic hyphema is a potentially sight-threatening condition. Principles of management are to exclude **life-threatening and other sight-threatening injuries, control intraocular pressure,** and **prevent corneal blood staining**. Management of the hyphema depends on the amount of hyphema, intraocular pressure, and duration. In this patient, in the absence of other injuries and contraindications, acutely I will treat the patient with **topical steroids** and **cycloplegics,** and **topical glaucoma medications** with oral acetazolamide and potassium cover with advice on posturing, complete bed rest, and risk of re-bleed. I will then monitor the patient closely and perform a gonioscopy after the hyphema clears to look for angle recession. Surgical indications would include **hyphema with intraocular pressures > 60 for one day or > 35 for seven days, early evidence of corneal blood staining, total hyphemas persisting for > five days or any hyphema that fails to resolve to < 50% by eight days. Patients with sickle cell hemoglobinopathies will require intervention if the pressure is ≥ 25 for 24 hours or if there are repeated spikes to > 30 for two to four days**.

Q Question 11.3 How will you Manage if the Patient then Develops Total Hyphema with IOP > 50 Uncontrolled for Seven Days?

Principles of management of hyphema:
- To prevent glaucomatous damage
- To prevent corneal blood staining
- To prevent formation of peripheral anterior synechiae

This patient is at risk of developing optic neuropathy and corneal blood staining. This is an indication for early surgical intervention. I will start the patient on tranexamic acid in the absence of contraindications. I will first attempt anterior chamber washout (AC maintainer, adrenaline in BSS infusion, aspiration with Simco) failing which I will then perform limbal delivery of the blood clot or automated hyphectomy with a vitrector. Long-term wise, I will perform gonioscopy to look for angle recession and monitor for glaucomatous damage.

Q Question 12 Viva Stem: How do you Manage Hyphema in a Patient with Neovascularization from Proliferative Diabetic Retinopathy (PDR)?

Management of this patient can be divided into **systemic and ocular** management. Systemically, I will co-manage with the internist to control his **vascular risk factors**. Ocular management will depend on patient factors including only eye, **high visual requirement**, and **presence of blood dyscrasias**, as well as **ocular factors which include intraocular pressures, duration**, and **amount of hyphema**, as well as **visual prognosis**. I will assess the visual potential by checking the visual acuity (assessing for light projection in all four quadrants if the vision is hand movement or worse) and relative afferent pupillary defect (by reverse method if obstructing the pupil) and perform a B scan to look for retinal detachments. If there is a view of the fundus, I will look for macula lesions, increased cup-disc ratio and retinal detachments. I will perform **urgent retinal photocoagulation** (especially to the superior retina as the superior view might be the best). For the hyphema, I will first manage conservatively, asking the patient to lie at a **posture of 45 degrees**, advice the patient to **rest in bed**, start the patient on **topical cycloplegics** and **steroids** in the absence of contraindications, and start the patient on glaucoma medications if intraocular pressure is raised.

Indications for surgical intervention include **persistent total hyphema with intraocular pressures more than 50 mmHg for more than five days, total hyphema that fails to resolve to less than 50%, pressures more than 25 mmHg for more than six days, persistent hyphema for more than nine days, or if the patient has Fuch's endothelial dystrophy or sickle cell anemia**. Other indications for early surgical intervention include presence of fundus abnormalities such as dense vitreous hemorrhage preventing laser photocoagulation or presence of retinal detachments.

(Other scenarios of DM with glaucoma include patients with poorly controlled DM 3/52 post-phaco coming in with BOV discomfort, IOP high: worried about NVG secondary to DR progression. Other causes include steroid response, retained nuclear fragments, uveitis reactivation, endophthalmitis, other previously undiagnosed glaucomas e.g. POAG; malignant glaucoma is less likely in a subacute scenario.)

Q Question 13 Viva Stem: How would you Manage a Four-year-old Child Presenting with Hyphema who has Symptoms of Eye Pain and Blurring of Vision?

Hyphema is a potentially sight-threatening condition, and management depends on the amount of hyphema, intraocular pressure, duration, and underlying cause. In a child, there is **concern about development of amblyopia as the hyphema obstructs the visual axis**. I will examine the patient's history for any **trauma** (especially keeping in mind non-accidental injuries), duration, progression of symptoms, and previous ocular or systemic conditions. I will also check to see if there is a family history of ocular disease. After excluding **life-threatening injuries**, I will assess the optic nerve function by checking the visual acuity by age-appropriate method, relative afferent pupillary defect by reverse method if the pupil is poorly reactive, color vision, and confrontational visual fields if possible. I will assess orbital injuries by checking for proptosis/enophthalmos, limitation of extraocular movements, and lid injuries.

If the child is cooperative, I will check the anterior segment under the slit lamp looking for signs of **globe rupture** and **assessing the amount of hyphema, intraocular pressure, anterior chamber activity, associated sphincter rupture, iridodialysis, cataract, or lens subluxation**. I will also look for signs of **uveitis such as band keratopathy and keratitic precipitates, examine the iris for rubeosis, tumors**, or yellowish nodules suggestive of **juvenile xanthogranuloma**. I will next perform a dilated fundal examination looking for **cup-disc ratio, optic nerve swelling, retinal tears or detachment**, or **dialysis or proliferative retinopathy such as familial exudative vitreoretinopathy** or **Coat's disease**.

If the child is uncooperative, I will do the examination under anesthesia and perform a gonioscopy, looking for evidence of rubeosis or tumors. In this patient, in the absence of other injuries and contraindications, acutely I will treat the patient with **topical steroids, cycloplegics, and topical carbonic anhydrase inhibitors** (paediatrics: alphagan is contraindicated as it causes respiratory depression; timolol might need punctal occlusion – consider CAI or xalatan as first line) while advising the parents on posturing, complete bed rest and risk of re-bleed (three–five days due to absorption of microclots). As hyphema involves the visual axis, there **is increased risk of amblyopia**. I will then **monitor the patient closely and consider early surgical intervention if improvement is slow**.

> **Q** **Question 14 OSCE Stem: Examination of Patient's Anterior Segment findings (see Figure 3.10).**

On examination of the patient's right eye, there is presence of **corectopia** inferior temporally with **ectropion uvea** from 6 to 9 o'clock of the pupil with associated **mid-peripheral anterior synechiae** at 5 to 10 o'clock. There are associated areas of **iris stromal atrophy** at 4 and 8 o'clock regions and **iris naevus** from 4 to 8 o'clock but no **pseudopolycoria**. There is no posterior embryotoxon and the anterior chamber is shallow. The corneal endothelial has a **hammered silver appearance** but otherwise the cornea is clear and there is no glaucoma drainage device present. Examination of the contralateral eye shows it to be normal. This patient has features of **iridocorneal endothelial syndrome**. My differential is posterior polymorphous corneal dystrophy. I will perform a gonioscopy to look for angle closure and peripheral anterior synechiae anterior to Shwalbe's line, check the intraocular pressure, and conduct a dilated fundal examination for increased cup-disc ratio. I will check the **endothelial cell count, corneal pachymetry and a Humphrey's visual field, specular microscopy (looking for dark-light inversion** – cells bright and edges dark), and examine the patient's history for monocular glare and diplopia.

Note: High peripheral anterior synechiae: as it is due to abnormal endothelial growing onto the iris and pulling it up.

Iridocorneal endothelial syndrome is an indication for primary tube implantation.

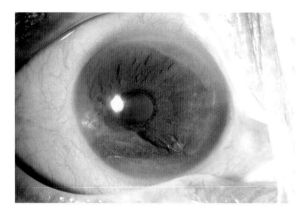

Figure 3.10 This patient has features of iridocorneal endothelial syndrome as correctopia, peripheral anterior synechiae and iris atrophy. It can be associated with complications such as corneal decompensation.

> **Q** **Question 15 OSCE Stem: Examination of Patient with the following Anterior Segment Signs (see Figure 3.11).**

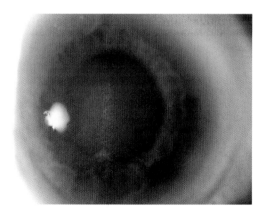

Figure 3.11 This sclerotic scatter photo shows the presence of Krukenberg spindle which is a classical feature of pigment dispersion syndrome.

On examination of the anterior segment, the patient was found to have features of **pigment dispersion syndrome** with the presence of **Krukenberg spindles** in the central corneal endothelium involving the visual axis. Otherwise the cornea is clear. The anterior chamber is **deep with posterior bowing of the iris** and **mid-peripheral iris atrophy**. The patient has a trabeculectomy bleb superiorly with a patent surgical iridectomy on retro-illumination. The bleb has a good height, normal vascularization with good posterior extent, and absence of scarring. Examination of the contralateral eye showed similar findings. There are **no other transillumination defects on retro-illumination**. I will check the intraocular pressure; perform a gonioscopy for **diffusely uniform hyperpigmented trabecular meshwork and queer iris configuration**; dilate the pupil to look for **Zentmayer's line at the equator of the lens**; examine the fundus for **increased cup-disc ratio** and **presence of lattice**, retinal tears, and detachments; check the refraction status; and perform a Humphrey's visual field test.

> **Q** **Question 16.1 Viva Stem: How do you Manage a Patient with IOP 25, Open Angles Normal CDR, Normal HVF?**

This patient likely has **ocular hypertension**. I will exclude other causes of raised intraocular pressure. I will examine the patient's history for blurring of vision, trauma, and use of steroids. I will also examine any significant past ocular history, as well as examine the patient's family history for glaucoma. I will check for visual acuity, relative afferent pupillary defect, the anterior segment for secondary causes such as pseudo-exfoliation or pigment dispersion. Risk of glaucoma progression in patients with ocular hypertension is low and management depends on patient and ocular factors. Patient factors include **age, life expectancy, family history of glaucoma**, and **visual potential of contralateral eye**. Ocular factors depend on **central corneal thickness (< 555), intraocular pressure, cup-disc ratio**, and **pattern standard deviation**. If the patient has significant risk factors for progression, I will start the patient on topical glaucoma medications in the absence of contraindications and monitor regularly with optical coherence tomography or Humphrey visual fields. (9.5% of untreated patients progress to POAG in an OHTS study.)

(Or question can be asked as raised IOP, what is the approach i.e. state that causes can be divided into open or closed angle, primary or secondary.)

> **Q** **Question 16.2 How do you Manage a Patient with IOP 15, Open Angles CDR 0.8 with Notching and HVF Defects?**

This patient likely has **normal tension glaucoma**. I will need to exclude other causes of optic neuropathy. I will take the patient's history of symptoms of **increased intracranial pressure such as headache, nausea, vomiting**, and **previous trauma, and examine**

whether there is any history of malignancy, migraines, obstructive sleep apnea, Raynaud's phenomenon, previous hypotension or surgeries requiring blood transfusion, or **steroid use,** as well as **history of refractive surgery which might affect pressure measurement**. I will assess the optic nerve function by checking the visual acuity, relative afferent pupillary defect, color vision, and confrontational visual field; check the anterior segment for other causes of open angle glaucoma such as pseudoexfoliation and pigment dispersion; and perform a dilated fundal examination for pallor more than cupping or thinned nasal rim that might suggest a compressive cause.

I will perform investigations, **phasing,** and optical coherence tomography, and check the central corneal thickness and Humphrey visual fields to look for location of defects. This patient is likely to have normal tension glaucoma, where risk of progression is low. Management depends on patient factors and ocular factors. Patient factors include age, life expectancy, family history of glaucoma, and visual potential of contralateral eye. Ocular factors depend on central corneal thickness, degree of cupping, and severity of visual field defects — whether field loss involves fixation and whether it is progressive (from the CNTGS trial for VF progression — decrease IOP by 30% decrease risk of VF progression from 35% to 12%). If there are significant risk factors, I will start the patient on topical glaucoma medications in the absence of contraindications, avoiding the use of beta blockers (mechanism of glaucoma 1; mechanical compression of ON sec high IOP 2; vascular component in NTG — it is thought to be vascular and hence beta blockers are avoided as we do not want further vasoconstriction and ischemia), and monitor the patient regularly.

Q **Question 16.3 Can you use Xalatan in a Patient with Uveitis?**

Prostaglandin analogues are **relatively contraindicated in patients with uveitis**. Hence, they are not the first-line treatment. However, if the patient has well-controlled inflammation and intraocular pressure control is suboptimal, prostaglandin analogues like Xalatan can be used with close monitoring.

Q **Question 16.4 When would you use Anti-Metabolites in a Trabeculectomy?**

In my center, **mitomycin C is routinely used in trabeculectomy due to high risk of scarring in our population**. However, general indications can be divided into patient and ocular factors. Patient factors include **young patient, previous failed trabeculectomy, pigmented race, patients on multiple topical glaucoma drops** or **known history of recurrent scars**. Ocular considerations include **neovascular, uveitic, congenital, aphakic, pseudophakic glaucoma, post-trauma,** and **iridocorneal endothelial syndrome**.

Complications of anti-metabolites divided into early and late stages.

Early	Late
Corneal epitheliopathy	Limbal stem cell deficiency
Anterior segment toxicity	Punctal stenosis (5-FU)
Glaucoma	Recurrent corneal erosion
Hypotony	Hypotony
Wound leak	Cataract
Infection	Toxicity to ciliary body and retina
	Bleb leak and infection (BRE, blebitis)
	Avascular bleb
	Scleral melt

Q **Question 17 OSCE Stem: Examination of Patient with the following findings (see Figure 3.12).**

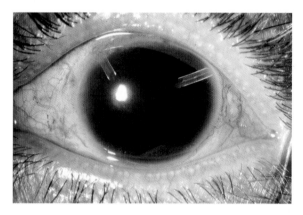

Figure 3.12 This young patient has bilateral congenital aniridia with associated congenital sensory nystagmus. He developed glaucoma in the left eye and underwent two glaucoma tube implantations for the treatment of his glaucoma.

On general inspection of the patient, there is **bilateral conjugate horizontal pendular nystagmus**. On examination of the left eye, there is **total aniridia** with presence of **two tubes** at 2 and 11 o'clock. The cornea is clear with **no signs of decompensation** or **scarring/pannus secondary to limbal stem cell deficiency**. There is no vitreous in the anterior chamber. The tubes are **well positioned**, not contacting the cornea, not extending into the visual axis and unblocked. The patient is phakic with a clear lens. The eye does not appear **bupthalmic**. On looking down, the bleb of the temporal tube is **well formed with normal vascularization** but the nasal bleb is **low with surrounding sub-Tenon's scarring**. There is **no extrusion or erosion** present. There is **no prior trabeculectomy** surgery as well. I will check the fellow eye, checking its visual acuity and intraocular pressure, conduct a gonioscopy to look for remnant iris stump, examine the fundus for increased cup-disc ratio, foveal or disc hypoplasia and chorioretinal colobomas, and take a family history and history of Wilms' tumor. This patient has bilateral aniridia with **associated secondary glaucoma requiring primary tube implantation** in the left eye.

Note: Inheritance: AD, AR, sporadic (WAGR syndrome).

In clinical cases with glaucoma tubes, it is important to state whether it is a primary or secondary implantation.

> Indications for tube implantation
>
> - Primary: for refractory glaucoma (i.e. conditions where trabeculectomy will likely fail) e.g. congenital glaucoma, aniridia, neovascular glaucoma, uveitic glaucoma, iridocorneal endothelial syndrome, trauma
> - Secondary: previous failed trabeculectomy

Q **Question 18.1 OSCE Stem: Examination of the Anterior Segment (see Figure 3.13).**

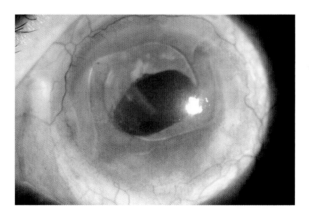

Figure 3.13 This patient, with a background history of poorly controlled diabetes, had a complicated ocular history beginning with a complicated cataract surgery requiring an ACIOL and vitrectomy with PFNO. His diabetic retinopathy subsequently progressed after the cataract operation, and he eventually developed neovascular glaucoma. A posterior chamber tube was implanted to control the intraocular pressure. He has corneal decompensation secondary to the ACIOL as well.

On examination of the left eye, there is presence of an angle supported anterior chamber intraocular lens that is well-centered with no phacodonesis and is associated with a superior temporal surgical iridectomy. The cornea is hazy with diffuse edema and guttata suggestive of corneal decompensation. The anterior chamber is deep and quiet with no vitreous in the anterior chamber but there is presence of heavy liquid inferiorly (not well seen in photo). The pupil is distorted but there are no dandruff-like fibrillary material along the pupil margin (that might suggest pseudoexfoliation syndrome as a cause for the complicated cataract surgery). The capsule is absent. There is presence of a posterior chamber tube (in this case it is difficult to differentiate whether it is suclus or pars plana tube) that extends into the visual axis and is unblocked. Examining superior nasally, the tube is well-covered with no extrusion or erosion and the bleb is well-formed with normal vascularization. There are no obvious rubeosis irides (as a cause for the tube implantation). The patient did not have a trabeculectomy surgery. I will check the visual acuity, relative afferent papillary defect, and intraocular pressure, conduct a gonioscoy, perform a dilated fundal examination for signs of previous retinal detachments (e.g. Scleral buckle indentation, retinopexy scars), and examine the fellow eye for risk factors for complicated cataract surgery (e.g. pseudoexfoliation syndrome, posterior polar cataracts). This patient probably had a right-sided complicated cataract operation with likely subsequent retinal detachment requiring the use of heavy liquid. The patient has likely developed secondary glaucoma requiring a primary tube implantation and also corneal decompensation. (This is just one possible scenario; the patient actually had a different history as narrated above.)

Q Question 18.2 What could Corneal Decompensation Result from?

The cornea could have decompensated secondary to a complicated cataract operation, glaucoma, or the presence of anterior chamber intraocular lens.

Q Question 18.3 Why was a Posterior Chamber Tube Inserted?

The posterior chamber drainage device was inserted due to anterior chamber crowding as a result of the presence of an anterior chamber intraocular lens as well as peripheral synechiae and to avoid further decompensation of the cornea. The patient likely has poor visual prognosis and thus the intraocular lens was not explanted.

Q Question 19 OSCE Stem: Anterior Segment of the Patient (see Figure 3.14).

On examination of the patient's right eye, there is presence of a superior **temporal laser peripheral iridotomy** that is **patent on retro-illumination** with areas of superior nasal **iris atrophy**. There are no other transillumination defects noted. There are also **several peripheral well-demarcated scars distributed circumferentially**, suggestive of previous **laser iridoplasty**. There is correctopia with the pupil deviated superior, and the patient is pseudophakic. The cornea is otherwise clear with no evidence of decompensation secondary to glaucoma. On downgaze, there is no evidence of **glaucoma**

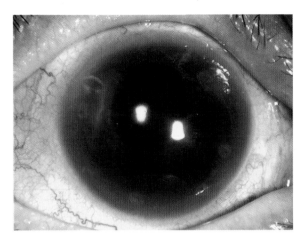

Figure 3.14 This patient had an acute angle closure episode which required iridoplasty and laser peripheral iridotomy to relieve the pupil block. The contralateral eye is shallow as well, with a patent peripheral iridotomy.

filtration surgery or drainage device implantation. On examination of the fellow eye, the patient is phakic with a nuclear sclerotic cataract, **shallow anterior chamber** with a patent superior temporal laser peripheral iridotomy, and no evidence of glaucoma filtration surgery or drainage device implantation. I will check the visual acuity, relative afferent papillary defect, and intraocular pressure, conduct a gonioscopy for narrow angles and areas of peripheral anterior synechiae, perform a dilated fundal examination for increased cup-disc ratio, and perform a Humphrey visual field. This patient is likely to have had previous acute primary angle closure in the right eye and primary angle closure suspect in the left eye.

> **Q** **Question 20.1 OSCE Stem: Examination of a Patient with the Following Signs (see Figures 3.15A–3.15C).**

On examination of the patient's left eye, there is presence of **fine to medium-sized pigmented stellate keratic precipitates diffusely** spread across the cornea. Otherwise the cornea is clear without evidence of corneal decompensation. The anterior chamber is deep and quiet with a white cataract and no obvious **phacodonesis**. The iris appears **moth-eaten and atrophic** without peripheral anterior synechiae, posterior synechiae, or Busacca or Koeppe nodules. On downgaze, there is absence of glaucoma filtration surgery or drainage device. The fellow eye appears normal, accentuating the **presence of heterochromia**. This patient has **Fuch's heterochromic iridocyclitis**. I will check the visual acuity with light projections, check the intraocular pressure, conduct a gonioscopy, check the **endothelial cell count, perform an anterior chamber tap, send for tetraplex cultures**, and **look for Amsler sign**.

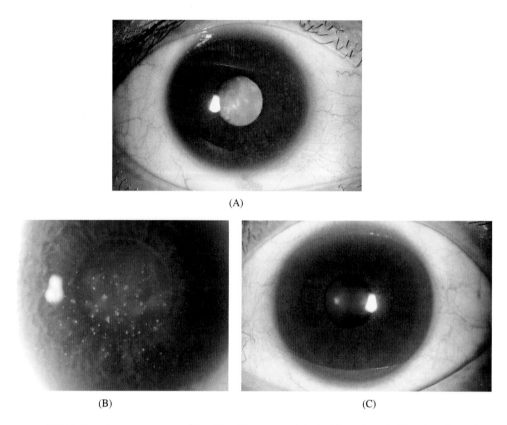

(A)

(B)   (C)

Figure 3.15 (A) Moth-eaten appearance of the iris with an associated white cataract. (B) Sclerotic scatter image highlighting the diffuse fine-medium stellate keratic precipitates. (C) Contralateral eye which is normal, highlighting the heterochromia of the iris when both eyes are compared. This patient has right Fuch's heterochromic iridocyclitis which is usually a unilateral disease.

Q Question 20.2 What are the Causes of Hypertensive Uveitis?

Causes can be divided into **viral**, such as varicella zoster, herpes simplex, and cytomegalovirus; **bacterial**, such as tuberculosis; **parasitic**, such as toxoplasmosis; **inflammatory**, such as sarcoidosis; and **masquerade** such as lymphoma.

Q Question 20.3 How would you Investigate a Patient with Hypertensive Uveitis?

I will exclude infective causes by performing an anterior chamber tap, sending for tetraplex for herpes, varicella, cytomegalovirus, and toxoplasmosis, as well as tuberculosis polymerase chain reaction. I will look for Amsler sign, order a chest X-ray, mantoux T spot/TB quantiferon, syphilis LIA IgM and IgG with VDRL, and assess for sarcoidosis by looking at chest X-ray for hilar lymphadenopathy and spiral computer tomography scans.

Management can be divided into **treating the intraocular pressure** and **treating the underlying condition**. I will co-manage the patient with the **uveitis and glaucoma team** and start the patient on glaucoma topical medications in the absence of contraindications, failing which I will consider glaucoma drainage implantation. If the underlying cause is infective, I will treat with anti-virals/anti-bacterials. If it is inflammatory, I will treat with topical steroids and keep in view immunosuppressants and systemic steroids.

Q Question 21 OSCE Stem: Anterior Segment Examination of the Following Patient (see Figures 3.16A and 3.16B).

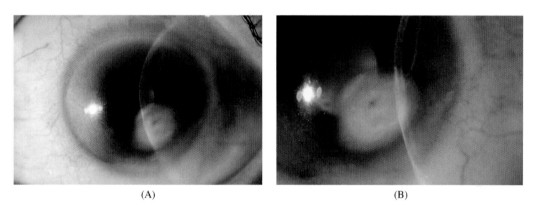

(A)   (B)

Figures 3.16A and 3.16B Peters anomaly. Note the iris adhesion to the area of the leukoma seen using the slit beam illumination.

On examination of the left eye, there is presence of a **well-demarcated deep stromal scar** located in the inferior temporal cornea not involving the visual axis. There is presence of **correctopia** with the pupil drawn toward the area of the scar. On casting a slit, there is **anterior synechiae with iridocorneal** touch at the area of the scar suggestive of a **leukoma**. Otherwise the anterior chamber is deep and quiet centrally. There is no obvious **posterior embryotoxon** or **iris atrophy** or **pseudopolycoria**. The patient is phakic with a mild nuclear sclerotic cataract. On retroillumination, there are no transillumination defects. On downgaze, there is no evidence of previous glaucoma filtration surgery or drainage device implantation. Examination of the fellow eye shows similar findings. This patient has **Peter's anomaly**. I will check the visual acuity and relative afferent papillary defect, conduct a gonioscopy, check the intraocular pressure, carry out a dilated fundal examination for increased cup-disc ratio, and examine systemically for **Peters plus syndrome** (short stature, cleft lips, mental retardation).

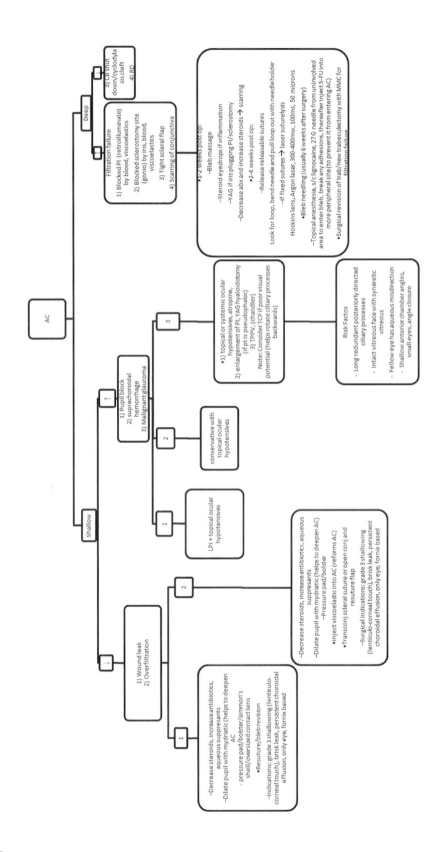

AC

Deep

Filtration failure
1) Blocked PI (retroilluminate) by blood, viscoelastics
2) Blocked sclerostomy site (gonio) by iris, blood, viscoelastics
3) Tight scleral flap
4) Scarring of conjunctiva

3) CB shut down/cyclodialysis cleft
4) RD

•1-2 weeks postop:
  –Bleb massage
  –Steroid eyedrops if inflammation
  –YAG if iris plugging PI/sclerostomy
  –Decrease abx and increase steroids → scarring
    •2-4 weeks post op:
    –Release releasable sutures
Look for loop, bend needle and pull loop out with needle holder
    –If fixed sutures → laser suturelysis
Hoskins lens, Argon laser, 300-400mw, 100ms, 50 microns
  •Bleb needling (usually 6 weeks after surgery)
–Topical anesthesia, s/c lignocaine, 27G needle from uninvolved area to enter bleb, break any adhesions, thereafter inject 5-FU into more peripheral site (to prevent it from entering AC)
  •Surgical revision of trab/new trabeculectomy with MMC for filtration failure

Shallow

1
1) Pupil block
2) suprachoroidal hemorrhage
3) Malignant glaucoma

3
•1) topical or systemic ocular hypotensives, atropine,
2) enlargement of PI, YAG hyaloidotomy (if pt is pseudophakic)
3) TPPV, (chandler)
Note: Consider TCP if poor visual potential (helps rotate ciliary processes backwards)

Risk Factos
- Long redundant posteriorly directed ciliary processes
- Intact vitreous face with syneretic vitreous
- Fellow eye has aqueous misdirection
- Shallow anterior chamber angles, small eyes, angle closure

2
conservative with topical ocular hypotensives

1
LPI + topical ocular hypotensives

↓
1) Wound leak
2) Overfiltration

2
–Decrease steroids, increase antibiotics, aqueous suppresants
–Dilate pupil with mydriatic (helps to deepen AC)
    –Pressure pad/bolster
•Inject viscoelastic into AC (reforms AC)
    –Transcon) scleral suture or open conj and resuture flap
–Surgical indications: grade 3 shallowing (lenticulo-corneal touch), brisk leak, persistent choroidal effusion, only eye, fornix based

1
–Decrease steroids, increase antibiotics, aqueous suppresants
–Dilate pupil with mydriatic (helps to deepen AC
  - pressure pad/bolster/simmon's shell/oversized contact lens
    •Resuture/bleb revision
–Indications: grade 3 shallowing (lenticulo-corneal touch), brisk leak, persistent choroidal effusion, only eye, fornix based

CHAPTER 4

VITREORETINA AND UVEITIS

Q **Question 1.1 Viva Stem: Describe the Photo in Figure 4.1.**

This is the limited retinal photo of the patient showing presence of a **horseshoe tear** with associated **retinal detachment**. I will check the rest of the fundus with a binocular indirect ophthalmoscope to determine the **location of the tear, size of the retinal detachment, involvement of the macula, presence of proliferative vitreoretinopathy,** presence of **other retinal tears,** and predisposing factors such as **lattice** and **myopic fundus.** I will examine the fellow eye, check the visual acuity and relative afferent pupillary defect, take the patient's history regarding duration of symptoms, trauma, refractive status, and any previous ocular surgeries, as well as investigate any family history of retinal tears or detachment.

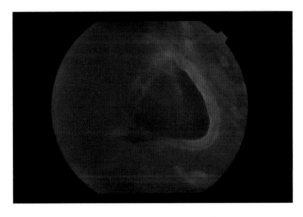

Figure 4.1   Horse shoe retinal tear.

Q **Question 1.2 What is Lincoff's Rule?**

Lincoff's rule is a **set of principles** to guide the **localization of retinal breaks** in patients with **primary rhegmatogenous retinal detachments.**

- For **superior** retinal detachments **crossing the midline,** the tears are localized to a **triangle bounded at the apex at the ora at 12 o'clock; at the base at the equator between 11 to 1 o'clock.**
- For **superior** detachments **not crossing the midline,** the break is within **1.5 clock hours from the superior edge of the subretinal fluid.**
- For **inferior** retinal detachments, the break is at the side with the **higher level of sub-retinal fluid.**
- For **inferior bullous** retinal detachments, the break is **superior to the horizontal meridian.**

Q **Question 1.3 How would you Manage this patient (Figure 4.1)?**

This is a sight-threatening condition and relative ocular emergency. Management depends on patient and ocular factors. Patient factors include fitness for surgery, ability to posture face-down, and need for air travel. Ocular factors include duration of symptoms, size of retinal tear, number and location of retinal tears, extent of retinal detachment, presence of tractional component, and pre-existing glaucoma. Options include barrier laser for limited retinal detachments, pneumoretinopexy, scleral buckling, or pars plan vitrectomy with gas or silicone oil.

Q **Question 1.4 When would you Perform Scleral Buckling?**

I will perform scleral buckling for a **young** patient with the following: **phakic, tears anterior to the equator, inferior tears localized to a single quadrant or multiple tears within the same meridian, retinal dialysis, no vitreous hemorrhage, tractional retinal detachment, giant retinal tear,** nor **proliferative vitreoretinopathy.**

Q **Question 1.5 When would you Perform Pars Plana Vitrectomy on a Patient with Retinal Detachment?**

I will perform vitrectomy for a patient who is **pseudophakic** and has **multiple tears not in the same meridian, posterior tears, giant retinal tears, traumatic retinal detachment, proliferative vitreoretinopathy, tractional retinal detachment** or with **vitreous hemorrhage, and macular hole retinal detachment.**

Note: traumatic GRT needs TPPV +/– SB with shallow indent; retinal dialysis needs SB +/– TPPV.

Q **Question 1.6 When would you Perform Subretinal Fluid Drainage?**

I will perform subretinal fluid drainage in patients who are **elderly** (reduced RPE pump function) with a history of **glaucoma** (with SB tightening, IOP will rise if SRF remains) or who has undergone **cataract surgery**. I will also perform the drainage for very **bullous retinal detachments**, especially **inferior bullous detachments**, detachments with **proliferative vitreoretinopathy** and **viscous fluid** or in patients where **no tears are identified or sealed** (unlikely RPE pump able to resorb).

Q **Question 1.7 When would you Perform Pneumoretinopexy and How would you Perform It?**

I would perform pneumoretinopexy if the tear is located in the **superior eight clock hours** (8–4 o'clock), if there are **single or few tears within a one-clock hour area**, and if there is **no proliferative vitreoretinopathy, no history of glaucoma, no need for air travel, no media haze** or **opacity**, and **absolute certainty of no other breaks**. I will perform the procedure under informed consent in the treatment room under sterile techniques with topical anesthesia, aiming to inject **1.2 mL of non-expansile gas**. I will inject **0.3 mL of neat (100%) C_3F_8 perfluoropropane** (0.6 mL SF_6 or 0.4 mL C_2F_6) through a **pars plana entry** aiming to inject into the **cortex** and forming a **single large bubble** (avoid fish egging). I will lay the patient **face down** first and gradually elevate the head in a **steam-roller technique**. I will feel the **digital intraocular pressure** and check for **spontaneous central retinal artery pulsation**. I will subsequently perform **retinopexy** or **transconjunctival cryotherapy** to seal the break.

Q **Question 1.8 How do you Perform Scleral Buckle Surgery?**

I will perform scleral buckle surgery with informed consent in the operating theater under regional anesthesia and in sterile conditions. I will first perform a 360-degrees conjunctival **peritomy** with clean dissection of tenons, **sling** the recti muscle using 2/0 silk sutures, identify and mark sites of break using indirect biomicroscopy with a 20 diopter lens with **indentation**, plan the site for subretinal fluid drainage, **pre-place the encirclage** (with or without segment), anchoring with 5/0 nylon, perform **subretinal fluid drainage** via cut down technique, refill the eye with air if it turns hypotonus, perform **cyrotherapy** followed by **tightening** of the sclera buckle, re-examine to ensure that the retinal tears are **supported,** check for **spontaneous central retinal artery pulsation** and **digital intraocular pressures**. If pressures are high, I will perform an **anterior chamber paracentesis**. I will then close the conjunctiva using 7/0 vicryl.

Q Question 1.9 What are the Complications of Scleral Buckle Surgery?

Complications of scleral buckle surgery can be divided into **intraoperative, early postoperative**, and **late postoperative** complications. Intraoperative complications include rectus muscle trauma, suprachoroidal hemorrhage, hypotony, vitreous or retinal incarceration, globe perforation (due to sclera sutures), buttonhole of conjunctiva, and raised intraocular pressure. Early postoperative complications include raised intraocular pressure, redetachment secondary to unidentified breaks, iatrogenic breaks, suprachoroidal or vitreous hemorrhage, and endophthalmitis. Late complications include anterior segment ischemia, strabismus, myopic shift or astigmatism, buckle intrusion/extrusion/migration/exposure, proliferative vitreoretinopathy, non-resolving subretinal fluid, and glaucoma (secondary to vortex vein compression).

Q Question 2.1 Viva Stem: What are the Principles of Vitrectomy for Diabetic Tractional Retinal Detachment and Indications for Diabetic Retinopathy?

Principles of vitrectomy for diabetic tractional retinal detachment would be to **segmentate** and/or **delaminate the fibrovascular tractional bands** followed by **endolaser, endodiathermy to achieve hemostasis** and **long-lasting tamponade** (in the presence of retinal break).

The common indications will include **tractional retinal detachment threatening the macular, combined tractional and rhematogenous retinal detachment**, and **persistent vitreous hemorrhage in patients with prior laser** (three months for type 1, six months for type 2).

Other Indications	
1.	Ghost cell glaucoma
2.	Persistent CSME with anterior posterior traction
3.	Anterior hyaloid fibrovascular proliferation
4.	Presence of rubeosis with vitreous hemorrhage preventing PRP
5.	Severe premacular hemorrhage

Q Question 2.2 When would you Perform Panretinal Photocoagulation for a Diabetic Patient?

I will perform panretinal photocoagulation when the patient has **proliferative diabetic retinopathy** as well as **severe non-proliferative diabetic retinopathy**, especially when the patient is **young**, has longstanding **type 2 diabetes** of **long duration, has poor glucose control**, has the **other eye blind from diabetic retinopathy, has a family history of** blindness, has **poor compliance to follow-up**, if the patient is going for **cataract operation,** or (if patient is female) she is **pregnant with gestational diabetes**.

Q **Question 2.3** When would you Perform a Fundus Fluorescein Angiogram for Diabetic Retinopathy?

Fundus fluorescein angiogram is indicated in diabetic retinopathy for **therapeutic** as well as **diagnostic purposes**. Indications include **differentiating intraretinal microvascular abnormalities versus neovascularization, determining the extent of ischemic maculopathy** and **peripheral capillary fallout, and delineating areas of leakage within the macula that is amenable for laser treatment.**

Q **Question 3.1** Viva Stem: Describe and Outline your Management of a Patient with Bilateral BOV (see Figures 4.2A and 4.2B).

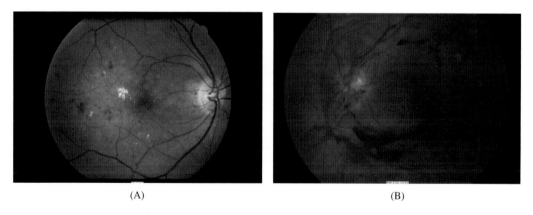

(A) (B)

Figure 4.2 (A) Right moderate non-proliferative diabetic retinopathy with clinically significant macula edema. (B) Left proliferative diabetic retinopathy with vitreous hemorrhage.

Figures 4.2A and 4.2B are the colored fundal photographs of both the patient's eyes. Figure 4.2B shows high-risk **proliferative diabetic retinopathy** in the left eye as evidenced by **extensive neovascularization of the disc** as well as **neovascularization elsewhere** nasal, superior, and inferior to the disc and along the superior temporal arcades with **fibrovascular proliferation** and preretinal hemorrhage superiorly and inferiorly but no **tractional retinal detachment**. There are also multiple **dot blot flame hemorrhages** distributed in all four quadrants and **venous beading**. The macula does not appear to be thickened but I will **confirm it under the slit lamp using a 78 diopter lens**. Cup-disc ratio is 0.4 and the disc is pink.

Figure 4.2A shows the right posterior pole with presence of dot and blot hemorrhages around the macula region with **cotton wool spots** temporally. There is absence of neovascularization at the disc or elsewhere in this photo. There are **hard exudates** concentrated temporal to the fovea extending to within 1 disc diameter from the fovea with macular thickening, but I will **confirm it under the slit lamp using a 78 diopter lens**. I will **examine the peripheries,** assess the **visual acuity,** check the **anterior segment for rubeosis** and **raised intraocular pressure,** perform a **gonioscopy,** check the **lens status** (as cataract might make PRP harder to perform), examine the patient's history for **duration of diabetes and control,** as well as concomitant vascular risk factors. In summary, this patient has left proliferative diabetic retinopathy without clinically significant macular edema and right **non-proliferative diabetic retinopathy** of **at least moderate severity** with **clinically significant macular edema.**

Management can be divided into **systemic** and **ocular** management. Systemically I will co-manage with the internist to control the patient's diabetes and vascular risk factors. Ocular management will depend on the stage and presence of clinically significant macular edema. For this patient, I will perform **urgent panretinal photocoagulation in the left eye, counseling the patient regarding the risk of worsening of macular edema with panretinal laser.** In the right eye, in the presence of **foveal** involving clinically significant macular edema, the mainstay of treatment is monthly intravitreal anti-vascular endothelial growth factor for at least six months; treatment should continue until the macula is dry or there is stabilization of macular edema and vision for two consecutive visits. If the macular edema is non-foveal-involving, I will treat with focal laser, targeting at microaneurysms in the macula amenable to laser therapy.

> **Q** **Question 3.2** How will you Differentiate Intraretinal Microvascular Abnormalities from Neovascularizations?

Intraretinal microvascular abnormalities are **flat, do not cross vessels, do not leak,** and are **connections between venules** and **arterioles;** they **stain on fundus fluorescein angiogram.** Neovascularisations are **raised vessels with leakage** and **crosses over other vessels;** they **exhibit leakage on fundus fluorescein angiogram.**

> **Q** **Question 3.3** How will you Perform a Grid Laser?

I will perform a grid laser with **informed consent** under **topical anesthesia** using the **argon laser** machine. I will sit the patient comfortably, and using a **Mainster focal lens** with a setting of **100 mW 100 microns 100 ms,** I will apply the **laser burns with a spacing of two spot sizes apart** (modified ETDRS guidelines) **at least 500 microns away from the fovea** and **500 microns from the temporal edge of the optic disc,** aiming for a **barely perceptible gray burn.**

I will perform panretinal photocoagulation with **informed consent**, under **topical anesthesia** using a **Volks quadrispheric lens** at the **argon laser** machine with settings of **200 mW 200 microns 200 ms**, aiming to put in **2000–3000 shots over two to three sessions**, titrating to achieve a **gray-white burn 0.5 to 1 spot size apart** (0.5 spot size for PDR, 1 spot size for SNPDR). I will first **demarcate my boundaries along the superior and inferior arcades, 500 microns nasal to the nasal edge of the disc and 2 disc diameters temporal to the fovea**. I will **treat the inferior retina first** before completing the superior portion.

Q Question 3.5 What are the Complications of Panretinal Photocoagulation?

Complications can be split into **early** and **late**. Early complications include **foveal** and **iris burns, vitreous hemorrahge, retinal tear and detachment,** and **worsening of macula edema**. Late complications include **constricted visual fields, reduced contrast** and **visual deterioration,** and **epiretinal membrane** and **choroidal neovascularization**.

Q Question 4 Viva Stem: Describe and Outline the Management of the Fundal Lesion (see Figures 4.3A and 4.3B) in this 60-year-old Patient.

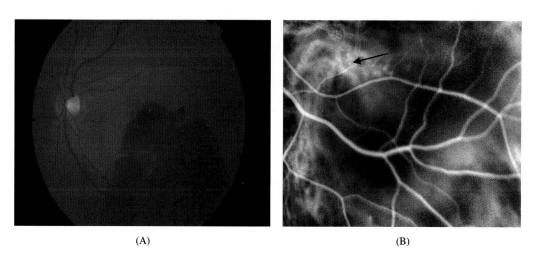

(A) (B)

Figures 4.3 (A) This patient has extensive subretinal hemorrhage with an orange nodule and absence of drusen suggestive of the presence of polypoidal choroidal vasculopathy. (B) Indocyanine green angiography with a cluster of grape-like hyperfluorescent spots and surrounding areas of blocked hypofluorescence due to the subretinal blood.

This colored fundal photograph of the patient's left eye (Figure 4.3A) shows **massive submacular hemorrhage** more than 6 disc diameter in size involving the fovea with an **extrafoveal orange nodule** 1 disc diameter inferior to the fovea. The subretinal blood extends beyond the inferior arcades. There is **absence of drusen**. This is suggestive of an **extrafoveal polypoidal choroidal vasculopathy**. The **indocyanine green angiography** image (Figure 4.3B) shows the presence of a **cluster of grape-like hyperfluorescent polyps** *(black arrow)* surrounded by areas of blocked fluorescence secondary to blood.

Management of polypoidal choroidal vasculopathy should be **individualized,** and depends on the **duration of loss of vision, size of the lesion, and location of the lesion**. I will examine the patient's history for **duration of symptoms, any prior treatment, smoking,** and **systemic co-morbids**. I will advise the patient to **stop smoking**. Treatment modalities include (1) **monthly intravitreal anti-vascular endothelial growth factors monotherapy in the absence of contraindications till the macula is dry** or (2) **combination of anti-VEGF with photodynamic therapy or focal laser therapy. I will explain to the patient regarding risks of treatment as well as retinal epithelium rip (PCV will require combination therapy with PDT).**

> **Q** **Question 5.1 OSCE Stem: Examination of Patient with the Lesion in Figure 4.4.**

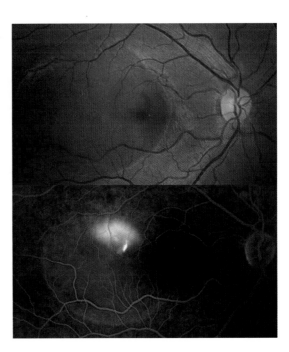

Figure 4.4 Right central serous chorioretinopathy seen in the fundal photograph. The fundus fluorescein angiography shows a characteristic focal hyperfluorescence with leakage in a smoke stack appearance suggestive of central serous chorioretinopathy.

On examination of the right fundus, there is a localized area of **subretinal fluid** about 5 disc diameter centered temporal to the fovea with no associated **pigment epithelial detachment**, no **subretinal blood**, and no **retinal pigment epithelium atrophy**. There is no associated **optic disc pit or optic disc coloboma**. This patient has a central serous chorioretinopathy of the right eye. I will check the **peripheries** (multifocal CSCR), check the **contralateral eye**, check the **visual acuity** and **relative afferent pupillary defect**, and examine the patient's **history** for **steroid** or **alternative medicine use**. I will also examine the patient's **psychosocial history**. Fundus fluorescein angiogram in the venous phase shows **pooling** of dye with an area of leakage with a **smoke stack appearance** about 1.5 disc diameter temporal to the fovea.

> **Q** **Question 5.2 What are the Indications for Treatment and How would you Treat?**

Indications for treatment include **high visual requirement, persistent central serous retinopathy for more than six months, recurrent central serous retinopathy with declining vision**, and **fellow eye also affected by central serous retinopathy with poor resultant visual acuity**. Treatment options include **focal laser** or **half fluence photodynamic therapy**.

> **Q** **Question 6 OSCE Stem: Examination of Patient with the Lesion in Figure 4.5.**

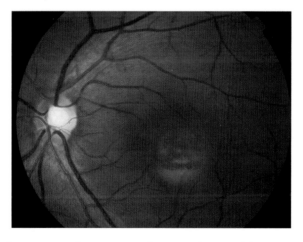

Figure 4.5 Left stage 3 Best disease with a pseudohypopyon.

On examination of the patient's left fundus, there is an **elevated subretinal area** well-circumscribed measuring 1.5 disc diameter in height and width associated with **vitelliform deposits** in a **pseudohypopyon configuration** involving the fovea and extending inferiorly. There is no **associated subretinal blood** or **retinal pigment epithelium atrophy**. The disc is pink, cup-disc ratio 0.5, and vessels are normal. I will examine the periphery for similar findings. On examination of the right eye, there is a **subretinal vitelliform lesion** in an **egg-yolk configuration** measuring about 1.5 disc diameter in height and width centered at the fovea. There is no associated **subretinal blood or fluid**. I will examine the periphery for similar findings and complete my examination by checking the **visual acuity** and **relative afferent pupillary defect** and **examining the family members**. This patient has Best's dystrophy with stage 3 on the right eye and stage 2 on the left eye. I will investigate by performing an **electroretinogram** which might be normal as well as an **electrooculogram which will show a decreased Arden's index < 1.5**. I will treat the refractive error (induced hyperopia from the swelling) and **monitor for development of choroidal neovascularization**.

Stage	Description
I	Previtelliform: normal vision, normal or only subtle RPE changes (tiny, central honeycomb structure centrally) with abnormal EOG.
II	Vitelliform: classic "egg-yolk" lesion. 30% have ectopic lesions. Normal vision or mild vision loss.
III	Pseudohypopyon: break through the RPE, layering of lipofuscin. Vision similar to stage II.
IV	Vitelleruptive: breakup of material with "scrambled egg" appearance. Vision may be similar or mildly decreased from stage I/II.
V	Atrophic: Central RPE and retinal atrophy. Vision may range from 20/30 to 20/200.
VI	CNV: This complication occurs in about 20% of patients. Vision often decreased to 20/200 or worse.

Q Question 7.1 Viva Stem: How would you Manage an 80-Year-old Wheelchair-Bound Patient with Good Visual Acuity in the Right Eye (VA 6/120 for 1.5 years) with Fundal Examination and Optical Coherence Tomography (see Figures 4.6A and 4.6B)?

Figure 4.6A is the fundal photograph of the right eye showing the presence of a **full-thickness macular hole** about 1 disc diameter in size with **yellowish deposits at the base, no posterior vitreous detachment**, and no **subretinal fluid**. This patient has a stage 3 full-thickness macular hole. The optical coherence tomography in Figure 4.6B shows the corresponding cross-sectional cut across the large full-thickness macula hole with associated **schitic changes** and no subretinal fluid. Management will depend on **patient and ocular factors**. This is an elderly female patient and **posturing** might be difficult (in view of her being wheelchair-bound). Her **visual requirements** might be low and she has good

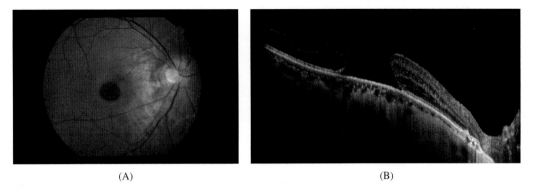

|(A)|(B)|

Figure 4.6 (A) The fundal photograph shows a large, full-thickness macula hole of about 1 disc diameter in size without surrounding subretinal fluid. (B) The optical coherence tomography of the same patient illustrates the full-thickness macula hole with rounding of the edges which suggests chronicity of the lesion.

vision in the contralateral eye. Ocular-wise, her prolonged blurring of vision and the stage 3 macular hole are **poor prognostic features**. I will counsel the patient and **manage conservatively**.

Q Question 7.2 What is the Staging for a Macula Hole?

A macular hole can be staged using the **Gass classification**.

Stage 1A	**Occult** macular hole with **foveal cyst, yellowish deposits,** and **absent foveal reflex**
Stage 1B	**Impending** macular hole with **centripetal spread of the yellowish deposits**
Stage 2	**Full thickness** macular hole **< 400 microns** with yellow ring of deposits
Stage 3	**Full thickness** macular hole **≥ 400 microns** with **subretinal fluid and yellowish deposits at the base**
Stage 4	**Full thickness** macular hole **≥ 400 microns** with **posterior vitreous detachment**

Q Question 8 OSCE Stem: Examination of a Patient with Fundal Lesion (see Figure 4.7).

On examination of the fundus, there is **thickening of the retina** with **cystoid changes in a cartwheel configuration** with a lamellar hole suggestive of **juvenile X linked retinoschisis**. The Watzke–Allen test is negative (could be associated with **diffuse granular appearance of the retinal pigment epithelium**). On examination of the peripheries, there are no associated **peripheral retinoschisis, vitreous veils,** or **retinal detachments**. Examination of the left fundus shows similar findings. In summary, this patient has features of juvenile X-linked retinoschisis. I will check the **visual acuity** and **relative afferent pupillary**

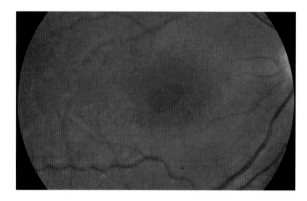

Figure 4.7 This young patient has bilateral thickening of the macula with a cartwheel appearance suggestive of X-linked retinoschisis.

defect, examine the **family members**, and perform an **optical coherence tomography** and **electroretinogram looking for electronegative B wave** (muller and bipolar). There is no definitive treatment available and management is **conservative**. I will also provide **genetic counseling** to the patient. (There are reports of clinical improvements with oral acetazolamides or topical dorzolamides.)

> **Q** Question 9 OSCE Stem: Examination of a Patient's Fundus (see Figure 4.8).

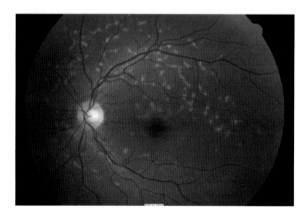

Figure 4.8 The presence of yellowish subretinal pisciform flecks involving the macula and peripheral retina is a classical feature of Stargardt disease. It is inherited in an autosomal recessive pattern — ABCA4 gene.

On examination of the left fundus, there is evidence of multiple **yellowish subretinal pisciform fleck-like deposits** involving the macula and posterior pole. The retinal pigment epithelium appears granular but there is no **Bull's eye maculopathy**. There is no subretinal fluid or blood to suggest presence of choroidal neovascularization. There is **no disc pallor and vessels are not attenuated**. On examination of the periphery, there is presence of **yellowish subretinal pisciform fleck-like deposits**. Examination of the right eye shows similar findings. This patient has **Stargardt disease** without Bull's eye maculopathy. I will check the **visual acuity** and **relative afferent pupillary defect**, examine the patient's **history for onset of visual loss**, check the **family members**, and perform a **fundus fluorescein angiogram to look for dark choroid** (diffuse dark choroid).

Note: OCT and AF can be offered for monitoring of progression, +/– ERG.

> Differentials to Bull's eye maculopathy: congenital e.g. rod cone dystrophy, cone dystrophy, cone-rod dystrophy, Stargardt disease, LCA, Bardet–Biedl syndrome; acquired e.g. chloroquine/hydroxychloroquine, tamoxifen, clofazimine, chlorpromazine.

Q Question 10.1 Viva Stem: 70-year-old Patient Presenting with Acute Blurring of Vision (see Figure 4.9).

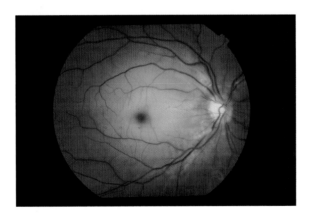

Figure 4.9 Right central retinal artery occlusion with the typical feature of a cherry red spot appearance.

This patient has a central retinal artery occlusion as evidenced by the **cherry red spot** and **pale retina**, and no **embolus is seen**. This is an **ocular emergency** and principle of management is to **re-establish retinal perfusion by dislodging the embolus**. I will take a quick patient's history regarding time of **onset of symptoms, cardiovascular risk factors** and check if the patient suffers from temporal headache or tenderness if no embolus is seen (or if there is a history of intravenous drug abuse in a young patient). I will check the **visual acuity, relative afferent pupillary defect,** and **intraocular pressure,** examine the rest of the **fundus for emboli**, and examine the **fellow eye**. I will check **systemically for carotid bruit, cardiac murmurs** (or temporal arteritis).

Management can be divided into **acute and chronic**. Acutely, I will ask the patient to breathe into a bag or inhale **Carbogen** (95% oxygen, 5% carbon dioxide); **lay the patient** down and **lower the intraocular pressure by performing ocular massage**; start **topical glaucoma medications** and **intravenous acetazolamide** in the absence of contraindications; and perform an **anterior chamber paracentesis** to lower the intraocular pressure (the principle being to increase the pressure gradient to dislodge emboli). For chronic management, I will co-manage with the internist to manage the patient's vascular risk factors. I will check the patient's blood pressure, fasting lipids and glucose (full blood count and ESR for giant cell arteritis), conduct 2D echocardiogram and carotid ultrasound to look for the source of emboli, and start the patient on anti-platelets after discussion with the patient's physician. I will monitor the patient subsequently for development of rubeosis.

Q Question 10.2 What are the Clinical Signs of Central Retinal Artery Occlusion?

Signs can be divided into **acute** and **chronic**. **Acutely**, the patient will present with very **poor visual acuity** with a **relative afferent pupillary defect**, associated **pale retina with a cherry red spot**, and **cattle trucking of the vessels**, as well as a **pale disc** and possible **presence of emboli**. At a **late stage** after perfusion, the main signs are **arteriolar attenuation, pale disc**, and possible **pseudo-retinitis pigmentosa changes in the periphery**. **Optical coherence tomography** will show **diffusely atrophic retina**.

Note: Features of central retinal artery occlusion on FFA — patchy choroidal flush (might have concomitant reduced ciliary artery flow due to vascular disease), increased arm retinal time, differential filling of arterioles, increased arteriovenous transit time.

Q Question 10.3 What are the Causes of Central Retinal Artery Occlusion?

The causes of central retinal artery occlusion can be divided into **systemic** and **ocular**.

Systemically, causes can be subdivided into thrombotic and embolic. Thrombotic causes includes vasculopathies such as diabetes and hypertension, vasculitis such as systemic lupus as well as giant cell arteritis, vasospastic causes such as migraine, coagulopathies such as anti-thrombin III, factor V leiden, homocysteinuria, protein C, and S deficiency, as well as hyperviscosity syndromes such as leukemia. Embolic causes include intravenous drug abuse, cardiac valvular disease or arrhythmias, and carotid stenosis and cosmetics such as filler injections.

Ocular causes include raised intraocular pressure such as post-gas or intravitreal injection.

Q Question 11.1 OSCE Stem: Examination of Patient with the following (see Figure 4.10).

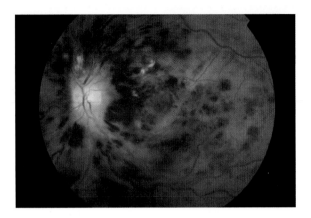

Figure 4.10 This patient, with a history of hypertension, developed left central retinal vein occlusion with a blood and thunder appearance. Presence of cotton wool spots suggests that this might be an ischemic central retinal vein occlusion.

On examination of the left eye, there are **dot blot** and **flame intraretinal hemorrhages** in all four quadrants associated with **cotton wool spots** and **dilated tortuous veins**. The disc is **swollen** with cup-disc ratio of 0.4 and associated **cystoid macula edema**. There is no **neovascularization of the disc or elsewhere**. This patient has central retinal vein occlusion. On examination of the contralateral eye, there is evidence of **hypertensive retinopathy** with silver wiring and arteriovenous nipping. I will check the **visual acuity, relative afferent pupillary defect**, and **intraocular pressure**; perform a gonioscopy to look for **nevoascularization of the angles**; examine the undilated iris to look for **rubeosis**; and check the patient's **blood pressure, fasting glucose**, and **lipids**. I will perform an **optical coherence tomography** and **fundus fluorescein angiogram** after the hemorrhages have cleared.

Q Question 11.2 Fundus Fluorescein Angiogram of Left Central Retinal Vein Occlusion. Please describe the findings.

This is the fundus fluorescein angiogram of the patient's left eye with views limited to the fundus. The **arm retinal time** is normal with arterioles well perfused at 6.7 s (normal 8–12 s) and there are multiple areas of **blocked fluorescence** secondary to the hemorrhages. (Comment on delayed **arteriovenous transit time** > 1 s after arterioles fill.) At 12.1 s there

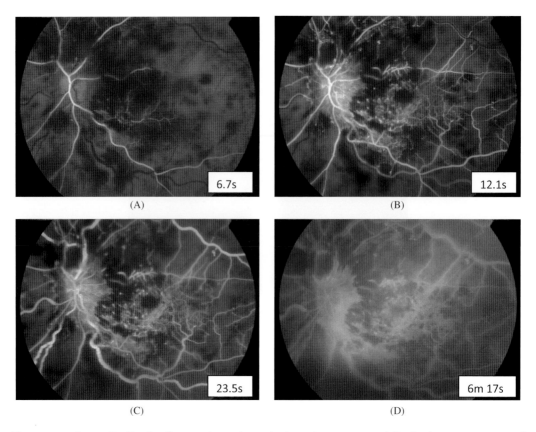

Figures 4.11A–4.11D Fundus fluorescein angiography is an important modality in the management of retinal artery occlusion. Note the presence of extensive capillary fallout, disrupted foveal avascular zone, and late leakage in the macula.

is **differential filling** of the inferior veins with **lamellar** flow in the superior veins. In the **peak venous phase at 23.5 s**, there is **capillary fallout** in the peripheries with **pruning of the capillaries** with an area of at least **10 disc diameter** with associated enlarged and disrupted **foveal avascular zone** (> 500 μm). In the late frames at 6 min 17 s, there is a **petaloid pattern of leakage in the macular**. There is no vessel wall staining secondary to vasculitis, no abnormal kink in the central retinal vein, and no evidence of **neovascularization at the disc or elsewhere**.

Q Question 11.3 How would you Manage this Patient?

Management can be divided into systemic and ocular. I will co-manage with an internist the patient's systemic vascular risk factors. Ocular management will depend on the **visual prognosis, degree of ischemia,** and presence of **macular edema**. I will perform baseline investigations such as **optical coherence tomography** and take fundal photographs. I will look at the peripheral views of the fundus fluorescein angiogram but it will likely be more than 10 disc diameters, suggestive of an ischemic occlusion (at least 10 DD for central retinal vein occlusion and 5 DD for branch retinal vein occlusion). I will monitor the patient closely and perform panretinal photocoagulation if rubeosis develops. However, if the patient has multiple risk factors or poor compliance to follow up, I will perform early pan-retinal photocoagulation. If there is significant cystoid macula edema, the mainstay of treatment is monthly intravitreal anti-vascular endothelial growth factor injection in the absence of contraindications, and I will treat until the macula is dry. Other options include intravitreal steroid injection.

Q **Question 11.4 What are the Side Effects of a Fluorescein Angiogram?**

The side effects of a fluorescein angiogram can be divided into mild or severe effects. **Mild** side effects include **nausea, vomiting, discoloration of the skin, tears and urine, pain over the injection side**, and **rashes**. **Severe** side effects include **bronchospasm, hypotension, cardiac arrest**, and **anaphylactic shock**.

Q **Question 12.1 Viva Stem: How will you Manage a 30-year-old Woman with Bilateral BOV, VA 6/24 (see Figures 4.12A and 4.12B)?**

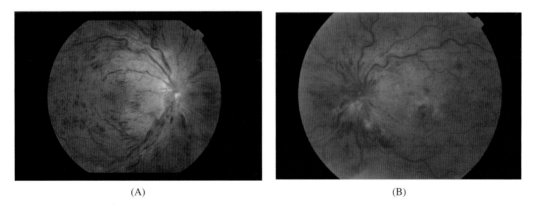

(A)   (B)

Figures 4.12A and 4.12B Patients with bilateral retinal vein occlusion should be investigated for vasculitis, hypercoagulable conditions and vasculopathy. In this case, this patient had a history of oral contraceptive pill intake which resulted in her hypercoagulable state.

This is the colored fundal photograph of the young patient showing bilateral central retinal vein occlusion right worse than the left. There are **dot blot** and **flame hemorrhages** in all four quadrants with **tortuous dilated veins** and **scattered cotton wool spots** with **blurred disc margins**. Cup-disc ratio is not discernable. The **macula looks edematous** but I will confirm this under the slit lamp with a 78 diopter lens. There are otherwise no **neovascularization of the disc or elsewhere**. I will check the **visual acuity, relative afferent pupillary defect**, and **intraocular pressure**, perform a **gonioscopy** for **neovoascularization of the angles**, examine the undilated iris for **rubeosis**, and check her blood pressure and fasting glucose and lipids. I will examine the patient's history for **vascular risk factors** and medication use such as **oral contraceptive pills**, and see whether she has a history of **coagulopathies** or **autoimmune conditions**. Management can be divided into systemic and ocular. I will co-manage with an internist systemically to assess her **vascular risk factors** and investigate for **immune conditions** or **hypercoagulable state** (such as multiple myeloma) and stop offending medications such as **oral contraceptive pills**. Ocular management will depend on the **visual prognosis, degree of ischemia**, and presence of **macular edema**. I will perform an **optical coherence tomography** as well as **fundal fluorescein angiogram** once the blood clears. If there is significant ischemia on the fluorescein angiogram, I will monitor the patient closely and **perform panretinal photocoagulation** if rubeosis develops. If there is significant **cystoid macula edema** with good visual prognosis, I will treat till the macula is dry, the mainstay of treatment being monthly intravitreal anti-vascular endothelial growth factor injections. If the visual prognosis is poor, I will offer conservative management.

> **Q** **Question 12.2 What are the Features to Look out for in the Fundus Fluorescein Angiogram for Branch Retinal Vein Occlusion?**

I will look out for increased **arm retinal time**, increased **arteriovenous transit time**; differential filling; **capillary non-perfusion** in the peripheries more than 5 disc diameter during the peak venous phase; increased or disrupted **foveal avascular zone**; early hyperfluorescence and late leakage indicative of **neovascularization** at the watershed area; petaloid late leakage in the fovea for **cystoid macular edema**; and **vessel wall staining** indicative of vasculitis.

> **Q** **Question 12.3 How would you Manage Branch Retinal Vein Occlusion?**

I will first take the patient's history of duration, progression, onset of BRVO, and **vascular risk factors** (or vasculitis in young patients or OCP). I will examine the anterior segment for **raised intraocular pressure**, examine the fundus for evidence of **sectoral flame** and blot hemorrhages with **tortuous** or **sclerosed veins** while looking out for the presence of **neovascularization** as well. I will take note of the **cup-disc ratio, hypertensive retinopathy,** and presence of **collaterals** or **vasculitis**; examine the macular for **cystoid macular edema**; and examine the fellow eye. Management can be divided into systemic or ocular. I will perform an **optical coherence tomography** and a **fundus fluorescein angiogram** to look for **capillary fallout and neovascularization**. Systemically, I will co-manage with an internist to control the **vascular risk factors**. Ocular management will depend on the **visual prognosis, degree of ischemia**, and presence of **cystoid macular edema**. If there is cystoid macular edema, I will treat till the macula is dry, the mainstay of treatment being monthly **intravitreal anti-vascular endothelial growth factor injections**. If there is development of neovascularization, I will start **sectoral retinal photocoagulation**. I will then monitor for development of complications such as **glaucoma** and **vitreous hemorrhage**.

> **Q** **Question 12.4** **What are the Causes of Poor Vision in Branch Retinal Vein Occlusion?**

The causes of poor vision include **macula edema, macula ischemia, vitreous hemorrhage, tractional retinal detachment,** and **neovascular glaucoma**.

> **Q** **Question 13** **OSCE Stem: Fundal Examination below.**

On examination of the patient's fundus, there is presence of **congenital hypertrophy of the retinal pigment epithelium** in the inferotemporal region as evidenced by a subretinal well-defined hyperpigmented lesion measuring about 4 by 4 disc diameter with **scalloped edges, halo along the edges,** and **areas of atrophic lacunae within the lesion**. I will examine the rest of the fundus and the fellow eye looking for similar lesions distributed with a **bear track appearance** and atypical features such as **fish tailing**. I will examine systemically for features of **type 2 neurofibromatosis** and refer the patient to a gastroenterologist to exclude **familial adenomatous polyposis (Gardner syndrome** or **Turcot syndrome)**.

> Gardner syndrome — osteoma. Turcot syndrome — medulloblastoma.
>
> Typical CHRPE is solitary or appears in groups, and is associated with neurofibromatosis type 2, incontinentia pigmenti, and golin gotze.
>
> Atypical CHRPE has oval fish tailing or hypopigmented polar bear appearance.

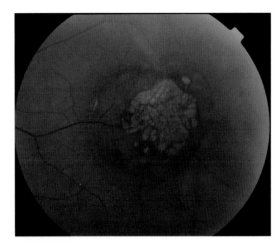

Figure 4.13 This patient has features of typical congenital hypertrophy of the retinal pigment epithelium. Risk of gastrointestinal track malignancies in this patient is low.

Q **Question 14 OSCE Stem: Examination of Disc Lesion.**

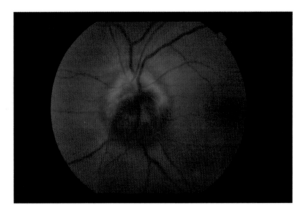

Figure 4.14 Optic disc melanocytoma.

On examination of the patient's fundus, there is melanocytoma at the optic disc as evidenced by a **dark pigmented lesion** with **feathered edges** extending from 4 to 8 o'clock of the optic disc and beyond the optic disc margin. There is no associated **subretinal fluid** or **subretinal blood** and there is an absence of **orange lipofuscin deposits**. The retinal vessels are normal and there is no **abnormal vascularization** over the tumor. I will examine the **peripheries** as well as the fellow eye, check the **visual acuity**, and perform a **B scan** and **Humphrey visual field** for visual field defects. I will take baseline photographs and follow up the patient regularly to look for enlargement and change in characteristics. (Note: Risk of malignant change is 1%.)

Q Question 15.1 OSCE Stem: Fundal Examination below.

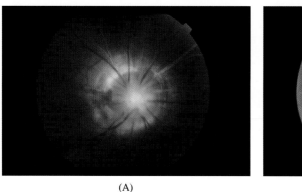
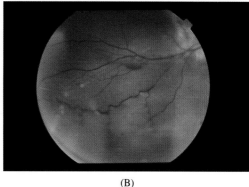

(A)   (B)

Figures 4.15   (A) A typical morning glory disc appearance. (B) Exudative retinal detachment.

On examination of the patient's fundus, there is presence of a **morning glory disc** as evidenced by a **large funnel shape excavated optic disc** with **overlying glial cells** and **surrounding chorioretinal pigmentation** associated with **supernumary straightened retinal vessels**. It is associated with inferior **retinal detachment** with a **smooth convex surface** extending from the inferior edge of the optic disc toward the periphery. I will examine the periphery for retinal breaks (absence of which supports diagnosis of exudative RD), examine the contralateral eye, and lay the patient supine to look for shifting fluid. I will check the **visual acuity** and **relative afferent pupillary defect**, examine the **oral cavity for basal encephalocele**, examine the patient's history for **recurrent strokes (Moyamoya disease)**, and check systemically for **PHACES syndrome**, and **frontonasal and septo-optic dysplasia**. (If associated with **pseudo-retinitis pigmentosa changes** extending from the disc edges, it could be suggestive of previous **exudative retinal detachment**.)

PHACES

Posterior fossa and other structural brain abnormalities

Hemangioma of the cervical facial region

Arterial cerebrovascular anomalies

Cardiac defects, aortic coarctation, and other aortic abnormalities

Eye anomalies

Sternal defects

Q Question 15.2 What would you Look out for when Performing an MRI for Morning Glory Disc?

I will look out for **basal encaphalocele** as well as **Moyamoya disease** affecting the circle of Willis and **dysgenesis of the posterior cranial fossa** in PHACES syndrome as well as **absent septum pellucidum**.

Q Question 16.1 OSCE Stem: Examination of Anterior and Posterior Segment.

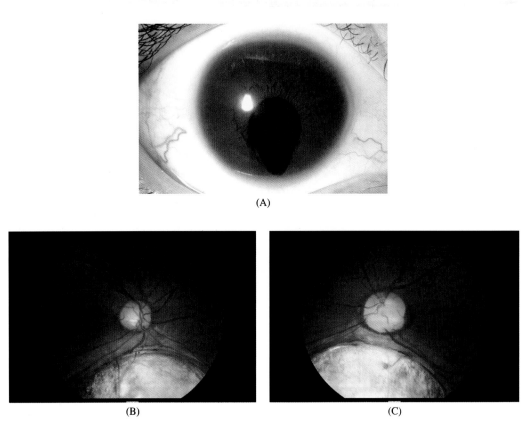

(A)

(B)　　　　　　　　　　　　　　　(C)

Figures 4.16A–4.16C Chorioretinal colobomas with associated key-hole iris coloboma. The inferior part of the left optic disc is involved as well.

On examination of the patient's red reflex, the patient has bilateral inferior iris defect with a **key hole appearance** due to **iris coloboma** without obvious lens coloboma. On examination of the right fundus, there is a large **chorioretinal coloboma** starting half a disc below the inferior border of the optic disc. It is excavated with pigmentation along the borders with baring of the underlying sclera, extending toward the periphery from 4 to

7 o'clock. There is no associated **exudative retinal detachment, pseudo-retinitis pigmentosa changes** or subretinal blood (CNV along the borders). Examination of the left fundus reveals similar chorioretinal coloboma but with an **associated optic disc coloboma** between 6 and 8 o'clock. I will check the **visual acuity**, and **relative afferent pupillary defect**, check the anterior segment under the slit lamp for lens **coloboma** as well as **posterior lenticonus** and **posterior embryotoxon**, examine systemically for **trisomy 13, 18, 22 and CHARGE syndrome**, and perform a **Humphrey visual field test**.

Q Question 16.2 What is the Pathology.

The underlying pathology is due to the **failure of closure of the embryonic fissure which occurs commonly inferior nasally**.

Differentials to macular coloboma
- North Carolina dystrophy type 3
- central choroidal atrophy
- central choroidal areolar dystrophy

CHARGE

Coloboma of the eye, central nervous system anomalies

Heart defects

Atresia of the choanae

Retardation of growth and/or development

Genital and/or urinary defects (hypogonadism)

Ear anomalies and/or deafness

Q Question 17   OSCE Stem: Examination of Bilateral Fundus (see Figures 4.17A and 4.17B).

On examination of this patient's right fundus, there are multiple **crystalline subretinal deposits** mainly located within the macula associated with an area of **retinal pigment epithelium atrophy** measuring 6 by 6 disc diameter centered at the fovea and surrounding the optic nerve head but no macula edema. Otherwise the disc is pink and not swollen with cup-disc ratio of 0.7, and vessels are not attenuated. Examination of the fellow eye shows similar findings. I would like to examine the peripheries to look for **vessel attenuation, crystalline deposits**, and **chorioretinal atrophy**; examine the anterior segment for **crystalline keratopathy** and **vortex keratopathy**; check the **visual acuity** and **relative afferent pupillary defect**; and examine the family members. I will examine the patient's history

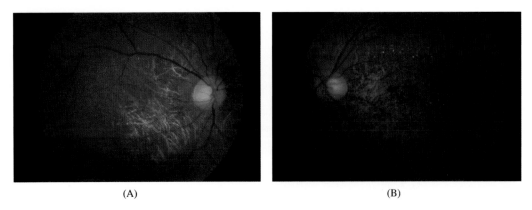

(A)   (B)

Figures 4.17A and 4.17B Bietti's crystalline retinopathy can result in progressive atrophy of the retina. In this patient, there are crystalline deposits mainly within the macula region with associated retinal pigment epithelium atrophy.

for **drug use** as well as **nyctalopia**. This patient is likely to have **Bietti's crystalline retinopathy**. Differentials include use of **tamoxifen, talcosis, oxalosis, cystinosis, methoxyflurane, nitrofurantoin**, and **autosomal dominant crystalline dystrophy** (other causes include PFT and familial autosomal drusen).

Crystalline
Retina

PFT
Betti
Cystinosis
Dsytrophy — AD crystalline dystrophy
Drugs — Tamoxifen/Talcosis/Canthaxanthin/Methoxyflurane/Nitrofurantoin
Gyrate atrophy

Q Question 18 OSCE Stem: Examine this Patient's Fundus (see Figure 4.18).

On examination of the fundus, the most obvious abnormality is the presence of retinal pigment epithelium **hyperpigmentation** temporal to the fovea with presence of **crystals** and **right-angled venules with grayish macula** and **loss of retinal transparency**. The fovea is dry without **cystoid macular edema** and **any signs suggestive of choroidal neovascularization such as subretinal fluid** or **blood**. I will examining the fellow eye, check the visual acuity, and perform an optical coherence tomography (looking for cystic

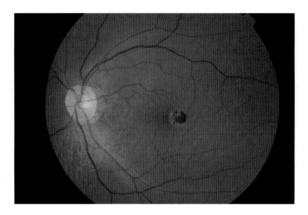

Figure 4.18 Another differential to crystalline retinopathy, this patient has type 2 parafoveal telangiectasia which is a bilateral disease.

spaces due to Muller cell degeneration). This patient has **stage 4, type 2 parafoveal telangiectasia**.

> **Q** **Question 19.1 OSCE Stem: Examine this Patient's Fundus (see Figures 4.19A and 4.19B).**

On examination of this patient's right fundus, there is a **pale disc** with a cup-disc ratio of 0.5 with associated **arteriolar attenuation** and **clumps of hyperpigmented bony spicules** in the posterior pole extending from the arcades toward the periphery. There is associated retinal pigment epithelium atrophy in the macula with **Bull's eye maculopathy** measuring 2 by 1.5 disc diameter centered at the fovea. There is **no epiretinal membrane**, and **no cystoid macula edema**. On examination of the optic disc, there is absence of **optic disc drusen** or **astrocytoma**. I will look at the peripheries for similar findings and exudation. Examination of the left eye shows similar findings. I will check the **visual acuity**; check the anterior segment for **keratoconus, glaucoma**, and **posterior subcapsular cataract**; check for systemic associations such as **deafness, cardiac abnormalities, ptosis and extraocular motility limitations, short stature, polydactyly, obesity, mental retardation**, and **ataxia**; and **check family members** as well. I will perform a **Goldmann visual field** and **electroretinogram**. This patient has bilateral pigmentary retinopathy secondary to advanced retinitis pigmentosa. Management will include **visual aids, referral to the society for the visually handicapped, monitoring and treatment of complications** such as cataract cystoid macula edema and epiretinal membrane.

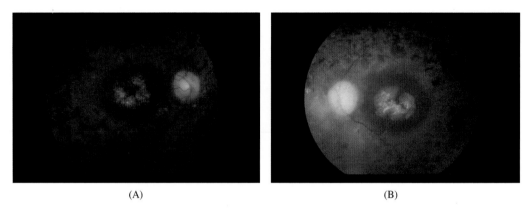

(A)   (B)

Figures 4.19A and 4.19B   A very common condition that appears in the exams, retinitis pigmentosa can lead to the development of Bull's eye maculopathy.

Q Question 19.2 What are the Risks of Cataract Surgery in Patients with Retinitis Pigmentosa?

I will counsel the patient regarding **guarded visual prognosis, significant postoperative glare**, and increased risk of **zonulysis** or **dropped nucleus**.

Q Question 19.3 If you were to Choose One Test, what would you Choose to Perform?

I would choose to perform an **optical coherence tomography** as it allows me to evaluate the **retinal pigment epithelium** and **ellipsoid zone of the foveal region** as well as **cystoid macula edema** and **epiretinal membrane**.

Q Question 20 Viva Stem: A 30-Year-old Patient Complains of Worsening Night Blindness. What are the Causes of Nyctalopia?

Causes of nyctalopia can be divided into stationary and progressive causes. The onset at this early age is likely progressive. Congenital causes of progressive nyctalopia can be classified as vitreoretinopathies such as Goldmann–Favre (enhanced S cone); retinal dystrophy such as retinitis pigmentosa, cone-rod dystrophies, Stargardt disease; choroidal dystrophy such as gyrate; and choroidemia. Acquired causes include vitamin A deficiency, cancer or melanoma-associated retinopathy, and other causes such as panretinal photocoagulation as well as use of pilocarpine eye drops for treatment of glaucoma.

Congenital		Acquired
Stationary	**Progressive**	**Acquired**
Normal fundus:	Vitreoretinal:	CAR
CSNB	Goldmann–Favre (enhanced S cone)	Vitamin A deficiency
		MAR
Abnormal fundus:	Retinal:	PRP
Oguchi, fundus albipunctatus	Cones, cone-rods, Stargardt, RP	Pilocarpine
	Choroidal:	
	Gyrate, choroidemia	

Q **Question 21 OSCE Examination: Patient with the following Fundal Features (see Figures 4.20A and 4.20B).**

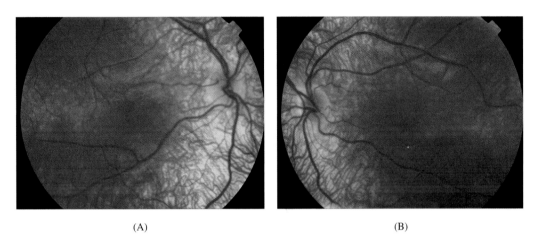

(A)   (B)

Figures 4.20A and 4.20B The pale hypopigmented fundus seen in these photos are classical of oculocutaneous albinism.

On general examination, the patient was found to have cutaneous albinism. On examination at the slit lamp, there is **poliosis of the lashes**. There is associated **pendular nystagmus**. On examination of the anterior segment, there is **depigmented diaphanous iris with transillumination defects**. There is **no associated Axenfeld anomaly**. On examination of the fundus there is presence of **optic** and **foveal hypoplasia** and a **depigmented diaphanous retina**. I will perform a **visual evoked potential** for **ocular misrouting** (even more crossed than uncrossed), the full blood count for **Chediak–Higashi** syndrome (raised WBC/leukemia) or **Hermansky–Pudlak** syndrome (thrombocytopenia), and examine for **sebaceous** and **basal cell carcinoma** and **solar keratosis**.

Note: Do remember to examine for systemic features of albinism.

Q Question 22 OSCE Examination: Fundus Examination Shown below (see Figures 4.21A and 4.21B).

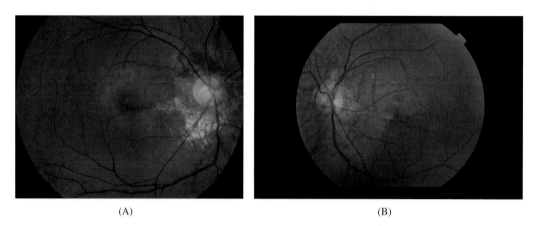

(A)   (B)

Figures 4.21A and 4.21B   Bilateral angioid streak with right choroidal neovascularization.

On examination of the patient's right fundus, there is presence of angioid streaks with multiple dark reddish well-defined **subretinal streaks** (break in Buch membrane) **emanating from the optic disc** toward the mid-periphery as well as the macula. There is **subretinal fluid** and **blood** with **involvement of the fovea**. There is no associated **optic disc drusen**. On examination of the peripheries, there is associated **peau d'orange retina** appearance in the temporal retina. Examination of the left fundus shows similar appearance but there is extension of the angioid streak toward the fovea with an area of retinal pigment epithelial atrophy with hyperpigmentation of about 3 by 3 disc diameter involving the fovea. There is no subretinal fluid or blood. This patient has angioid streaks with right secondary choroidal neovascularization. I will check for features of **Marfan** and Ehlers–Danlos syndromes such as subluxed lens as well as join hyperlaxity, stick plucked chicken skin appearance associated with **pseudoxanthoma elasticum**, history of **metastatic breast cancer**, and **sickle cell anemia**.

> **PEPSI**
>
> **P**seudoxanthoma elastica
> **E**hlers–Danlos
> **P**aget's disease
> **S**ickle cell
> **I**diopathic

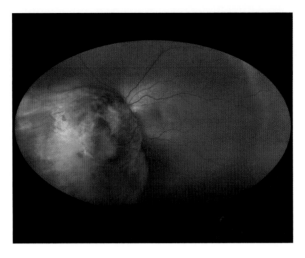

Figure 4.22 This Optos image shows a large choroidal melanoma obscuring the optic disc.

This is the colored fundal photograph of the left eye showing a **large subretinal pigmented mass lesion** inferonasally partially obstructing the view of the disc with **irregular edges** and possible superior **subretinal fluid** with associated **lipofuscin** and **absence of drusen**. There are **no satellite lesions** and **the vitreous is clear**. It is likely a **choroidal melanoma**. Differentials include metastatic tumor. I will check the rest of the fundus with **indentation**, check the fellow eye, check the visual acuity, relative afferent papillary defect, and anterior segment, and conduct a **gonioscopy** for extension as well as intraocular pressure.

Ocular melanoma is both **sight-** and **life-threatening**. The principles of management of ocular melanoma are to first **save life, then save the eye, and lastly, maximize visual potential** (similar to retinoblastoma). Factors to be considered can be divided into patient and ocular. Patient factors include patient's **fitness for systemic therapy, visual potential of contralateral eye**, and **systemic metastasis**. Ocular factors include **size, location**, and **extent** (any extrascleral or anterior spread), as well as **vision** and **presence of complications**. Systemically, I will co-manage with an oncologist and radiation therapist. For the ocular management, if the tumor is large as defined by more than **16 mm in diameter** or more than **10 mm in thickness**, I will offer the patient **enucleation**, especially if the patient is fit, has poor vision in that eye, and there is an absence of systemic metastasis and presence of anterior segment invasion. If the tumor is small as defined by a **diameter of 16 mm** or less and **thickness of 1.5–2.4 mm**, I will offer **local therapy such as focal laser photocoagulation, cryotherapy, plaque radiotherapy**, or **transpupillary thermal therapy (TTT)**. If the location is in an unfavorable location such as macular involving or peripapillary, I will observe the patient. If the tumor is **medium-sized** as defined by a **diameter of 16 mm or less** and a **thickness of 2.5–10 mm**, mode of treatment is controversial. I will offer the patient enucleation versus plaque radiotherapy (plaque radiotherapy saves the eye but not life). Other modalities include systemic chemotherapy, extenteration for extensive tumor, and external beam radiotherapy.

Q Question 23.2 What are the Poor Prognostic Features of Ocular Melanoma?

Poor prognostic features include histology that is predominantly **epithelioid cells (versus spindle A and B), genetics with gain of chromosome 8 and loss of chromosome 3, large size** (especially if thick or > 1 cm³ in volume), **anterior** or **extra scleral extension, recurrence**, or **systemic metastasis**. (Always think about size, location, and extent.)

Summary of the results of the Collaborative Ocular Melanoma Study

Small 1.5–2.4 mm Apical Height 5–16 mm Diameter	Medium 2.5–10 mm Apical Height ≤ 16 mm Diameter	Large > 10 mm Apical Height > 16 mm Diameter
21% grew by two years 31% grew by five years Factors associated with growth includes initial thickness and diameter, absence of drusen, presence of lipofuscin pigments	No clinical or statistical difference in survival rates between I_{125} brachytherapy versus enucleation up to 12 years after treatment	No difference in survival rates between enucleation alone versus enucleation with prior radiation Age and largest basal diameter of the tumor are the main factors affecting prognosis

Note: Conclusion form COMS Study

Medium: radiation versus enucleate

Large: enucleate (no need radiation prior)

Survival curve post-enucleation: Bi-modal (first peak a few years after surgery as a result of tissue handling during surgery, second peak is attributed to recurrence of the melanoma)

Q Question 23.3 What are the U/S Features of Melanoma?

The **A scan** characteristics include **high anterior surface spike with subsequent decremental low internal reflectivity with a cascading effect**.

On the **B scan, high anterior reflective surface** can be seen with a **homogenous hyporeflective core in a dome-shape/collar stud appearance** extending into the vitreous with associated **choroidal excavation, posterior acoustic shadowing**, and possible extension into the orbit with associated retinal detachment (might see flickering response in the mass secondary to pulsation of the supplying blood vessels). (When describing a mass on histo or B scan, mention large or small, whether there is extension to anterior segment/ lens or optic nerve and associated complications like RD.)

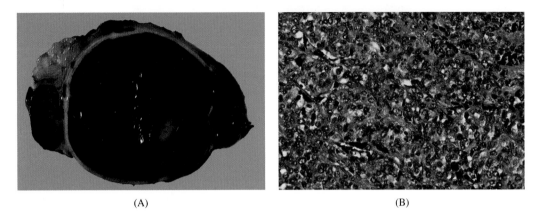

(A)   (B)

Figure 4.23 (A) Choroidal melanoma. Cut surface of an eye showing near-complete replacement by a tumor with brown-black coloration. The tumor fills the posterior and anterior chambers and has invaded through the sclera to form an extrascleral nodule posteriorly (left side of image). (B) Choroidal melanoma. The tumor cells have large irregular nuclei, many with prominent nucleoli. Finely granular brownish pigment can be seen in the cytoplasm of some cells (haematoxylin and eosin stain, original magnification x200).

Figure 4.23A is the cross section of a **gross specimen** of an **enucleated eye**. There is a **large brown black tumor** within the vitreous cavity that nearly occupies the entire eye. There is **extrascleral extension** of the tumor posteriorly. Figure 4.23B shows the histology under **high magnification**. The cells have an **epithelioid appearance, large irregular hyperchromatic nuclei** with **intracellular brownish pigment accumulation**, and **loss of differentiation** as well as **irregular arrangement**. These are features consistent with malignant melanoma with extrascleral extension which carry a poor prognosis.

Q **Question 24.1 Viva Stem: How do you Manage a Patient Complaining of Blurring of Vision and Floaters (see Figure 4.24)?**

This is the fundus photograph of the patient's left eye showing retinitis involving zone 1 as evidenced by large patch of **pale yellow lesion with fluffy edges** extending from the inferior pole of the optic disc down along the inferior temporal arcade. There is **sheathing** of the vessels, blot and flame hemorrhages with **cheese and ketchup appearance** in a perivascular **brush fire distribution** with foveal involvement. The **media** otherwise is **clear** without significant vitritis. This patient likely has **cytomegalovirus retinitis**. I will check the **peripheries** and the **contralateral** eye, check the **visual acuity, relative afferent pupillary defect,** and **intraocular pressure,** look in the **anterior chamber for activity,** and

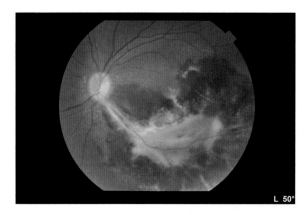

L 50°

Figure 4.24 This patient has cytomegalovirus retinitis involving the zone 1 region. It has the typical cheese and ketchup appearance with a perivascular distribution. This patient will require systemic and intravitreal treatment.

examine the patient's history for **immunocompromised states** such as steroid use or retroviral infections. I will check for **retroviral infections, CD4 count,** and **polymerase chain reaction of the blood for cytomegalovirus DNA** (for systemic cytomegalovirus retinitis), and performing an **anterior chamber aqueous tap for tetraplex** and **quantitative polymerase chain reaction**. Differentials include progressive outer retinal necrosis and toxoplasmosis chorioretinitis.

> **Q** **Question 24.2 How would you Manage a Patient with Posterior Capsular Rupture, and Who is CMV Positive and HIV Positive, and has a CD4 Count of 40?**

Cytomegalovirus retinitis is a **sight-threatening condition** and carries a guarded prognosis. Management can be divided into systemic and ocular. Systemically, I will co-manage the patient with the **infectious disease department** and **start the patient on highly active anti-retroviral therapy when the retinitis is quiet to avoid immune reconstitution uveitis**. Ocular management will depend on the **severity, location, and CD4 count**. Treatment options include intravitreal injections, vitreous implants, and systemic anti-virals. This patient has retinitis involving zone 1 area. I will start the patient on induction **intravitreal ganciclovir 2 mg in 0.04 mL twice a week for three weeks in the absence of contraindications, then switching to 2 mg in 0.04 mL once a week for maintenance**. Second-line treatment includes forscarnet or cidofovir. I will also start the patient on systemic intravenous **ganciclovir 5 mg/kg twice a day for two weeks, then 5 mg/kg once a day for maintenance**. Conversely, I can start the patient on **valganciclovir 900 mg twice a day for two weeks induction, then 900 mg once a day for maintenance**. I will treat the patient till the patient is immunocompetent (CD4 > 200). I will monitor the patient for immune reconstitution uveitis, uveitis secondary to drugs (e.g. cidofovir), and development of retinal holes or detachment.

Caution: Generally do not start HAART therapy until cytomegalovirus retinitis is treated, as it can cause CMO which is recalcitrant to treatment, and the patient may lose vision due to the CMO secondary to immune reconstitution uveitis.

Note: zone 1 is 1DD from disc and 2DD from fovea; needs systemic and IVT anti-viral while other zones need systemic therapy

Q **Question 25.1 OSCE Stem: Examine the Patient below (see Figure 4.25).**

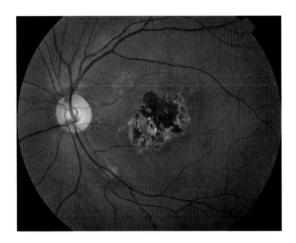

Figure 4.25   Left toxoplasmosis macula scar.

On examination of the left fundus, there is a large pigmented **macular scar** centered at the fovea measuring 1.5 disc diameters in width and 1.5 disc diameters in height with areas of **chorioretinal atrophy** and **absence of subretinal fluid** or **blood**. There is no **chorioretinitis**. This is likely a **toxoplasmosis scar**. Otherwise the vitreous is clear, cup-disc ratio is 0.5, and optic disc is **neither swollen nor hyperemic**, indicating there is no **vasculitis**. On examination of the peripheries, it is otherwise normal. Examination of the contralateral fundus shows it to be normal. I will check the **visual acuity** and the anterior segment for **keratic precipitates** and **anterior chamber activity**. Differentials include post-trauma, laser injury, macula coloboma or choroidal neovascularization.

Q **Question 25.2 How do You Manage a Patient who Presents with Eye Pain and Blurring of Vision?**

Figures 4.26A and 4.26B are the fundal photographs of the patient's left eye, showing a **pale whitish yellow area** measuring 2 by 2 disc diameter centered at the fovea with **fluffy**

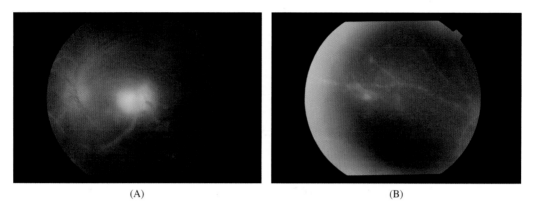

(A)	(B)

Figure 4.26 (A) Toxoplasmosis reactivation with severe vitritis obscuring the view of the fundus. It has a headlight-in-the-fog appearance. (B) Arteritis with a Kyrieleis' pattern.

ill-defined edges with overlying **media haze (likely vitritis)** and absence of associated scar. There is **optic disc swelling** with superior and inferior **arteritis in a Kyrieleis' pattern**. This is likely **primary toxoplasmosis chorioretinitis** (if it is adjacent to a scar, it will be reactivation of ocular toxoplasmosis). I will examine the periphery for other lesions; check the **visual acuity** and **relative afferent pupillary defect**; examine the **anterior segment for activity, granulomatous changes**, and **posterior synechiae**; and examine the **fellow eye**.

> **Q Question 25.3 How would you Manage?**

Management can be divided into patient and ocular factors. Patient factors include **immunocompromised patients** or **pregnant patients**. Ocular factors include **large lesions more than 1 disc diameter, lesions close to optic disc, papillomacular bundle or macula**, and **significant vitritis and cystoid macular edema**, or **complications like epiretinal membrane** and **tractional membrane**. I will start the patient on **triple therapy including sulfadiazine, pyrimethamine with folic acid, and steroids** in the absence of contraindications, failing which I will add sulfamethoxazole trimethoprim or clindamycin.

Note: The patient can be given piramycin if she is pregnant. Other options include atovaquone and azithromycin. Systemic steroids are contraindicated in AIDS patients.

> **Q Question 25.4 What are the Features of Toxoplasmosis in Acquired Immune Deficiency Syndrome (AIDS)?**

Features include **multifocal lesions, bilateral, not confined only to posterior pole, more severe inflammation, not adjacent to scar, requiring lifelong treatment**, and **involvement of central nervous system**.

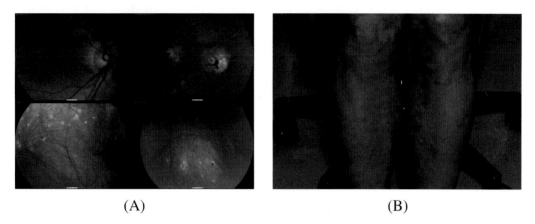

(A) (B)

Figures 4.27A and 4.27B Chronic Vogt–Koyanagi–Harada disease results in a sunset glow fundus and Dalen–Fuchs nodules in the periphery. They are associated with integumentary signs such as vitiligo that occurs late after the acute phase.

On general examination, the patient has **vitiligo, alopecia, and poliosis**. (Tips: Observe the patient as a whole to pick up tell-tale signs; do not rush in to examine the eye.) On examination of the right fundus, there is diffuse **retinal pigment epithelial atrophy** with a **sunset glow fundus appearance**. The **disc is not hyperemic or swollen**, cup-disc ratio is 0.6, and the disc has surrounding peripapillary atrophy. There is loss of the foveal reflex but no **subretinal fluid** noted. There is no **vitritis**. Examination of the periphery reveals focal areas of **pigmented chorioretinal atrophy suggestive of Dalen–Fuchs nodules**. Examination of the contralateral eye reveals similar findings with a pigmented macula scar measuring 1 by 1 disc diameter centered at the fovea with no subretinal fluid or blood, likely due to **secondary choroidal neovascularization**. This patient is likely to have Vogt-Koyanagi–Harada disease. I will check the **visual acuity, relative afferent pupillary defect**, and **intraocular pressure**, and check the **anterior segment for granulomatous inflammation** and **cataracts**. I will examine the patient's history for **trauma** or **ocular surgeries**, **tuberculosis, syphills, tinnitus, vertigo** or **deafness**, symptoms of **meningism like nausea, vomiting, headache, neck stiffness**, and **abdominal pain**.

Q **Question 26.2 How would you Manage this Patient?**

This patient is in the **chronic phase**. I will need to determine whether there is any activity and exclude other causes. I will like to investigate by checking the **chest X-ray, mantoux** and **syphilis VDRL LIA IgG IgM**, performing a **fluorescein angiogram looking for**

leakage (starry sky appearance only in acute stage) and **disc leakage or staining**, **indocyanine green angiogram** looking for **early phase choroidal patchy hyperfluorescence, mid phase fuzzy hyperfluorescence and leakage form the choroidal vessels, mid phase dark dots in the periphery** (granuloma) and **disc leakage or staining**. I will perform an **optical coherence tomography with enhanced depth imaging** looking for **choroidal thickening or atrophy** (and subretinal fluid if picture is acutely SRF +++, and B scan if acute to look for thickened choroid and to exclude posterior scleritis). I will refer to the **otolaryngologist for audiometry** to look for **high tone sensorineural hearing loss**, refer to the **neurologist for lumbar puncture** to look for **pleocytosis** (MS — pleocytosis, miller fisher — cytoabuminogenic dissociation). Management depends on the activity and fitness for **systemic immunosuppression**.

Q **Question 26.3 How would you Treat a Patient who presents Acutely with SRF?**

I will admit the patient for **intravenous steroids** in the absence of contraindications with subsequent conversion to oral steroids and steroid-sparing immunosuppressants. The patient will need **prolonged treatment up to a year** before stopping.

Q **Question 27 OSCE Stem: Examination of Patient with the following Fundal Lesion (see Figures 4.28A and 4.28B).**

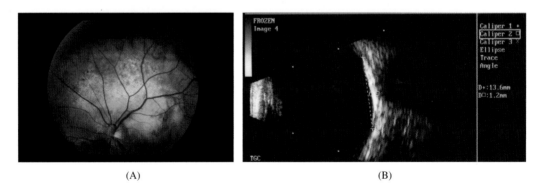

(A)　　　　　　　　　　　　　　　　(B)

Figures 4.28A and 4.28B Choroidal osteoma with a characteristic B scan with a pseudo-optic disc appearance.

On examination of the left fundus, the most obvious abnormality is a large **whitish subretinal** lesion measuring about 4 by 6 disc diameter located in the superior

peripapillary region surrounding the optic disc from 9 to 3 o'clock. There are areas of **clacification** within the lesion and the edges are **scalloped** with pigmentation. There is no subretinal fluid or blood (can be associated with CNV). The lesion extends into the macula but spares the fovea. This patient has **choroidal osteoma**. Differentials include **amelanotic naevus, choroidal metastasis**, or **choroidal hemangioma**. (B scan shows a **hyperreflective** layer with **posterior acoustic shadowing** creating a **pseudo-optic disc** appearance.)

Q Question 28 OSCE stem: Examination of Fundus (see Figures 4.29A and 4.29B).

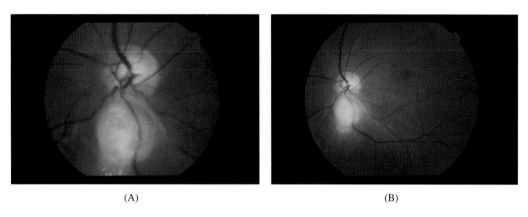

(A)   (B)

Figures 4.29A and 4.29B   Incidental left retinal astrocytoma.

On examination of the left fundus, the most obvious abnormality is the presence of a **yellowish mulberry-like intraretinal lesion** measuring about 1 by 1.5 disc diameters extending from the inferior pole of the optic disc, likely to be a **retinal astrocytoma**. There is **no surrounding subretinal fluid or blood**. There is absence of associated hypopigmented lesions and the disc is pink, not swollen, with a cup-disc ratio of 0.7. Otherwise the fundus is unremarkable with no associated nevi. I will examine the rest of the fundus for similar lesions, examine the anterior segment for features of **neurofibromatosis type I** such as lisch nodules and ectropion uvae, and hypopigmented iris lesions seen in **tuberous sclerosis**, examine the fellow eye, examine the patient systemically for neurofibromatosis type I and tuberous sclerosis, and examine the patient's history for mental retardation, seizures, and family inheritance.

Note: Classical triad of tuberous sclerosis — mental handicap, epilepsy, and adenoma sebaceum. Chromosome 9, AD inheritance.

Skin	CNS	Ocular	Visceral
Adenoma sebaceum	Astrocytic harmatoma	Retinal astrocytoma	Kidney — angiomyolipoma
Ash leaf spots	• Epilepsy	Hypopigmented iris	Heart
Shagreen patches	• Mental handicap	and fundal lesions	Subungal
Café au lait spots	• Hydrocephalus		
Skin tags	Cortical tubers		

Q. Question 29.1 OSCE Stem: Examination of Patient with Fundal Lesion (see Figure 4.30).

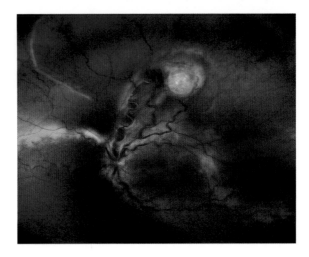

Figure 4.30 This Optos image provides an excellent view of a large left retinal capillary hemangioma with associated prominent feeding and draining vessel.

On examination of the left fundus, the most obvious abnormality is the presence of a **large circumscribed lesion** measuring **4 by 5 disc diameters, 5–6 disc diameters superior to the superotemporal arcades**. The lesion is **intraretinal, yellowish,** and **raised** with associated **tortuous feeding arteries** and **draining veins** with surrounding localized **subretinal fluid superiorly** but no blood or hard exudates. This is likely to be a **retinal hemangioma**. There are no scars to suggest **previous laser treatment**. There are no significant hypertensive retinopathy changes. The disc is pink and not swollen (for malignant hypertension from phaeochromocotyoma or papilloedema from central nervous system hemangioblastoma). I will examine the rest of the fundus with **indentation** to check for **other retinal haemangiomas,** check the fellow eye, and assess the visual acuity. I will examine the patient systemically for features of **von Hippel–Lindau syndrome**.

Note: Chromosome 3, AD inheritance. (Way to remember: VHL — 3 letters, for chromosome 3).

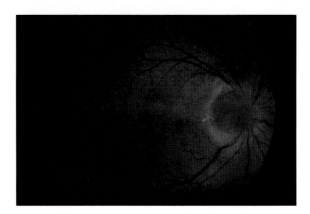

Figure 4.31 Optic disc capillary hemangioma.

I will investigate by performing a fundus **fluorescein angiogram** for **early hyperfluorescence** and **late leakage** as well as **optical coherence tomography** for subretinal fluid. If there are multiple lesions, I will **co-manage with an internist** to investigate for von Hippel–Lindau syndrome. As the lesion still appears **active**, I will treat **with focal laser photocoagulation to the lesion** and **the feeding vessel** (aim to blanch the feeding vessel). Other options include **intravitreal anti-vascular endothelial growth factor or photodynamic therapy or cyrotherapy**.

Note: Other rarer forms include peripapillary angioma.

Q **Question 30.1 OSCE Stem: Examination of the Anterior and Posterior Segment (see Figure 4.32).**

On examination of the patient's right posterior pole, there is presence of a **silicone oil reflex**. The posterior pole is **flat** with normal disc and cup-disc ratio of 0.4 and normal vasculature. There is a localized scar **superior nasal to the disc likely from a previous drainage retinotomy**. On examination of the peripheries, the retina is **flat** with presence of **uniform 360 degrees scleral buckle indentation** (i.e. only encirclage without segmental buckle) with **360 degrees** of **retinopexy/cryopexy scar posterior to 360 degrees retinectomy**. On examination in downgaze, there is **full fill** of the vitreous cavity with silicone oil. There are **no signs of emulsification**. This patient is likely to have had **previous rhegmatogenous retinal detachment complicated by proliferative vitreoretinopathy**. On examination under the slit lamp, the patient is **pseudophakic with a posterior chamber**

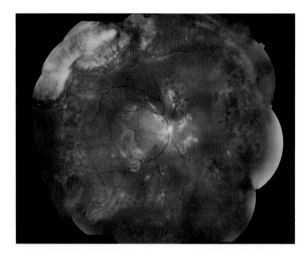

Figure 4.32 Right retinal detachment with proliferative vitreoretinopathy treated with scleral buckle, silicone oil peripheral iridectomy, and 360-degrees barrier retinopexy with retinectomy.

intraocular lens with an intact capsular bag. There is absence of an inferior peripheral iridectomy. The anterior chamber is otherwise **deep and quiet**. I will check the visual acuity, relative afferent pupillary defect, and intraocular pressure. I will also examine the fellow eye for **risk factors** for retinal detachment such as myopia and lattice degenerations.

Note: Keep a look out for retained subretinal silicone oil/heavy liquid which could be present in similar cases.

If a tear is seen, do comment on whether it is supported by the buckle.

> **Q** **Question 30.2 What is the Indication for Ando's Peripheral Iridectomy, and What is the Refractive Change Due to Silicone Oil?**

Ando's peripheral iridectomy is sited inferiorly as a prophylaxis toward secondary angle closure secondary to pupil block from the silicone oil which floats. In a patient who is aphakic, the anterior surface of the silicone oil forms a convex surface resulting in a myopic shift, while in a patient who is phakic, the anterior surface forms a concave surface resulting in a hyperopic shift.

> **Q** **Question 30.3 What is a Likely Cause of the Retinal Detachment in this Patient and Why?**

The retinal detachment likely occurred after cataract surgery with subsequent development of proliferative vitreoretinopathy. This is due to the presence of a posterior chamber intraocular with an intact capsular bag and no Ando's peripheral iridectomy (if retinal detachment with proliferative vitreoretinopathy occurred first, TPPL would have been performed with creation of an Ando's peripheral iridectomy with subsequent ACIOL or sutured PCIOL inserted).

Note: There are several possibilities and it depends on how the candidate argues. Another possible scenario could be the patient first developing primary RRD → SB+TPPV → cataract formation requiring surgery → redetachment with PVR — TPPV with SO.

Q **Question 31.1 Viva Stem: Describe the Photograph shown in Figure 4.33.**

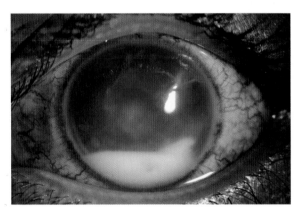

Figure 4.33 A classical presentation of endogenous endophthalmitis with an injected eye, fibrin, and hypoypyon with no view of the fundus.

This is the anterior segment photograph of the patient's left eye. The most obvious abnormality is the presence of **hypopyon** with a level approximately a quarter of the corneal height. This is associated with **conjunctival injection** and **hazy cornea with anterior chamber fibrin**. There are no obvious signs of **trauma** or **surgical scars**. This patient likely has **endogenous endophthalmitis**. I will check the **visual acuity, light perception** in all four quadrants if it is limited to hand movement or worse, **relative afferent pupillary defect**, and **intraocular pressure**. I will conduct a dilated fundal examination and examine the fellow eye. If there is no view, I will perform a **B scan** to look for **vitritis, choroidal abscesses**, and **retinal detachments**. I will take the vital signs and examine the patient **systemically for sources of infection**. I will next examine the patient's history for duration of pain; blurring of vision and redness; systemic features of infections such as fever, chills, and abdominal pain; any recent **ocular surgeries** or **trauma**, and any incidences of **immunocompromised states**.

Q Question 31.2 How would you Manage this Patient with No History of Ocular Surgery or Trauma?

This patient has endogenous infective endophthalmitis which is an **ocular emergency**. I will inform patient of the **guarded prognosis**. Management can be divided into **systemic** and **ocular**. I will **admit** the patient and perform an **urgent vitreous tap** and **injection of antibiotics** — **vancomycin 1 mg in 0.1 mL and ceftazidime 2.25 mg in 0.1 mL** in the absence of contraindication. I will send the tap for **microscopy** and **cultures**. I will then start the patient on systemic **intravenous ciprofloxacin 400 mg twice a day** and **intensive fortified topical antibiotics such as cefazolin** and **gentamicin**.

I will next perform investigations to localize the source. I will send off blood samples for **full blood count** (looking for raised total white blood cells and neutrophils), **erythrocyte sedimentation rate, C-reactive protein, liver function test, blood cultures**, and **urine for cultures** and **microscopy**. I will order **imaging tests** which include **chest X-ray, two-dimensional echocardiogram**, and **ultrasound of the hepatobiliary system**. I will co-manage the patient with the **infectious disease department** and trace the microscopy and cultures urgently over the next few days. I will **review the patient daily** for worsening or improvement, keeping in view repeat intravitreal injections after 48 hours. If retinal detachment develops or vision and inflammation continue to worsen, I will consider the patient for a pars plana vitrectomy.

Note: For post-cataract operation exogenous endophthalmitis, management depends on visual acuity. LP or worse requires immediate tap and jab and trans pars plana vitrectomy. If there is presence of retinal detachment, it is an absolute indication for trans pars plana vitrectomy.

Q Question 31.3 How will you Perform a Vitreous Tap and Jab and When will you Repeat It?

I will perform a vitreous tap and jab under **informed consent in the treatment room in sterile conditions and under regional anesthesia**. I will **prepare my culture plates and glass slides**, antibiotics such as **vancomycin 1 mg in 0.1 mL** and **ceftazidime 2.25 mg in 0.1 mL** in the absence of contraindications. I will use a **23G** needle attached to a **10-mL syringe, guard at 10 mm** from the tip with artery forceps, enter through a **pars plana site** (4 mm posterior to the limbus) directing it toward the center of the globe, **aspirate 0.2 mL of vitreous**, sending off for **cultures** and **gram stain**. I will next **inject the antibiotics** using a **27G** needle through a separate site. The procedure can be repeated after 48 hours.

Q Question 31.4 If there is a Dry Tap, what will you do?

If the tap is dry, I will reposition the needle. If it is still dry, I can attempt from a separate site and use a 21G needle, failing which I will refer the patient to the vitreoretinal surgeon for a diagnostic vitrectomy. (Do not give the jab if a tap is not done as it will raise the intraocular pressure and increase risk of central retinal artery occlusion.)

Q Question 32 OSCE Examination: Patient with the following Fundal Findings (see Figure 4.34).

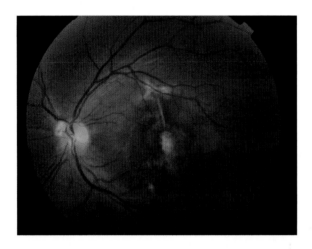

Figure 4.34 This patient sustained a blunt injury to the left eye with a resultant choroidal rupture. Unfortunately, the choroidal rupture involves the fovea, and a secondary choroidal neovascularization developed and left a scar.

This is the fundal photograph of the patient's left eye, showing a **curvilinear subretinal pale streak concentric to the optic disc** involving the fovea stretching around 3–4 disc diameter in length. There is an area of subretinal fibrosis about 0.5 disc diameter in size involving the fovea with no subretinal blood or fluid. This patient has choroidal rupture with evidence of previous choroidal neovascularization. The disc is pink and not swollen, and the rest of the fundus is flat. I will examine the peripheries for retinal tears or detachment. I will assess the **optic nerve function** by checking the **visual acuity, color vision, relative afferent pupillary defect,** and **confrontational visual field**; check for previous **orbital injuries** like lid laceration; check for other **ocular injuries** like previous globe rupture, iridodialysis, and subluxed cataract; check the **intraocular pressure**; and examine the **fellow eye**. I will examine the patient's history for the **injury** and **its mechanism**.

Note: If it is an acute presentation, check for life-threatening injuries and ask for loss of consciousness.

Q Question 33.1 Viva Stem: What would you Examine in a Patient who presents with Blurring of Vision, Floaters, and Recent Facial Rash?

I will first examine the patient's history for the **onset and duration** of the **blurring of vision, presence of pain**, and **photophobia**, as well as when the **rashes** occurred, distribution of the rash, and any **immunocompromised state**. I will check the **visual acuity** and **relative afferent pupillary defect**; check externally for **facial scars from previous vesicular rash**, check the **anterior segment for injection** and **scleritis, dentritic ulcer or geographical ulcer**, and **interstitial/stromal/disciform endothelitis**; check the **corneal sensation, anterior chamber activity and keratatic precipitates, intraocular pressure, posterior synaechiae**, and **cataract**; and perform a **dilated fundal examination** for **vitritis, vasculitis, acute retinal necrosis**, or **progressive outer retinal necrosis and optic neuritis**.

Q Question 33.2 Examination of the Fundus Reveals.

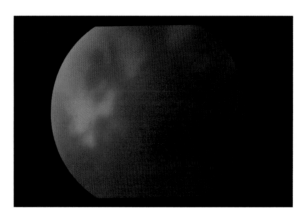

Figure 4.35 Patch of retinitis in a patient with acute retinal necrosis. Note that the media is hazy due to the presence of significant amount of vitritis.

This photo shows the superior retina of the patient's left eye showing multiple patches of retinitis as evidenced by **pale whitish yellow intraretinal lesions with fluffy ill-defined edges**, distributed **circumferentially** with **sheathing** of the **vessels** (usually arteritis but media haze makes identification of vessels difficult). The areas of retinitis involve the **anterior** retina and does not appear to encroach posteriorly, but I will examine the rest of the fundus to confirm, in the meantime looking for **retinal holes/tears** or **detachment**. The **media is hazy**, suggestive of the **presence of vitritis**. I will examine the optic disc and macular for swelling, examine the anterior segment for keratic precipitates and activity, check the visual acuity and relative afferent papillary defect, and examine the contralateral eye. This patient has **acute retinal necrosis**. (Progressive outer retinal nercrosis will have clear media without vitritis, minimal sheathing, involvement of posterior pole, and a cracked-mud appearance.)

Q Question 33.3 How would you Manage?

Acute retinal necrosis is a **sight-threatening condition** and carries a **poor prognosis**. I will examine the patient's history for duration of symptoms, recent systemic infections, and immunocompromised state. I will confirm the diagnosis by performing a **diagnostic aqueous tap**, sending for **tetraplex polymerase chain reaction** and especially looking for **herpes simplex** or **zoster virus**. Management can be divided into systemic and ocular. Systemically, I will co-manage with the **infectious disease department** and work up for **immunocompromised state** in patients with PORN. Ocular treatment will involve systemic medications such as **intravenous acyclovir 10–15 mg/kg three times a day** for at least **10–14 days** followed by **oral acyclovir 800 mg five times a day** in the absence of contraindications. Alternatives include **valacyclovir 1–2 g three times a day**. I will inject intravitreal **forscanet 2.4 mg in 0.1 mL** into the patient, consider starting systemic steroids early (after 48 hours), and monitor for response and development of retinal holes, tears, or detachment.

Summary of the Different Anti-Virals Used in Acute Retinal Necrosis (ARN)

	Systemic					Intravitreal	
	Acyclovir	Ganciclovir	Valacyclovir (Valtrex)	Famciclovir	Valganciclovir	Foscarnet	Ganciclovir
Dose	IV 10–15 mg/kg TDS daily 10–14 days, → 400–800 mg 5x/day 6–8 weeks	IV 5 mg/kg BD for 2 weeks → OM maintenance	1–2 g TDS for 6–8 weeks	500 mg TDS for 12 weeks, followed by taper for 13 weeks	900 mg BD for 3 weeks → 900 mg OM for 2 weeks before switching to oral acyclovir	2.4 mg/ 0.1 mL intravitreal as initial treatment	2 mg in 0.04 mL 2x/ week for 3 weeks → 1x/week maintenance
Use	Current standard		Emerging standard because of comparable AUC but lower peak concentrations, which translates to safer profile	Acyclovir resistance	Substitute to existing regimen	Especially when systemic treatment is contra- indicated	
Adverse effects	CNS toxicity: lethargy, delirium, seizures, renal failure		Hemolytic uremic syndrome, thrombotic thromboycytopenic purpura (in immuno- compromised patients > 8 g/day)	Minimal Similar to placebo	Myelotoxicity, sterility, CNS abnormalities		

Q **Question 33.4 What is the definition of Acute Retinal Necrosis?**

According to the American Uveitis Society, there should be at least **one area of retinal necrosis in the periphery, circumferential spread, rapid progression in the absence of anti-viral therapy, vitritis or anterior chamber activity,** and **peripheral occlusive arteriolitis**.

CHAPTER 5

NEURO-OPHTHALMOLOGY

1. Optic Disc and Optic Neuropathies

Q **Question 1.1 Viva Stem: How would you Manage a 30-Year-old obese woman who complains of Intermittent Blurring of Vision and Headache?**

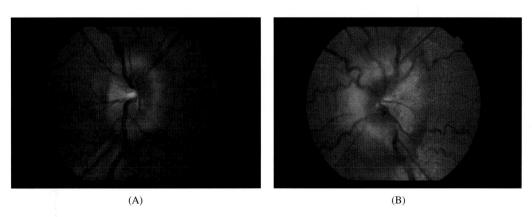

(A)   (B)

Figures 5.1A and 5.1B This patient presents with bilateral disc swelling secondary to idiopathic intracranial hypertension. It is important to exclude life-threatening causes of papilloedema as idiopathic intracranial hypertension is a diagnosis of exclusion.

This is the disc photo of both the patient's eyes, showing **bilateral disc swelling with hyperemia**. The overlying vessels are **tortuous** and **partially obscured** with concentric **Patton's line** seen in the left eye. The peripapillary retina otherwise appears normal, but I will examine the macula and rest of the fundus.

I will exclude **life-threatening causes** of bilateral disc swelling such as papilloedema from **raised intracranial pressure secondary to space-occupying lesion, dural venous sinus thrombosis, malignant hypertension,** or **meningitis**. Other causes of bilateral disc swelling include **idiopathic intracranial hypertension, hereditary optic neuropathies, toxic neuropathy** (less likely due to presence of headache; nutritional cause is unlikely as its onset is chronic), **bilateral consecutive optic neuritis, consecutive ischemic optic neuropathy, compressive lesions, infiltrative optic neuropathy,** and **pseudopapilloedema**. **Intraorbital causes** include severe thyroid eye disease and orbital inflammatory disease. **Intraocular causes** include bilateral consecutive retinal vein occlusion, posterior uveitis, or posterior scleritis.

I will examine the patient's history for symptoms of **transient visual loss**, duration of **onset and progression, headaches, nausea, vomiting, postural dependence**, presence of **tinnitus, diplopia, any fever or neck stiffness, systemic vascular risk factors** such as hypertension and previous **malignancies**; enquire for a **family history** of ocular disease; and examine the patient's **drug history** such as the use of oral contraceptive pills.

I will assess the **optic nerve function** by checking the **visual acuity, relative afferent pupillary defect, color vision,** and **confrontational visual fields,** especially taking note of **enlarged blind spots** and **visualizing the optic nerves**. I will check the pupils for **anisocoria** and **extraocular movements,** looking for **false localizing signs** and checking the patient's **contiguous cranial nerves**. I will perform a **Hertel's exophthalmometer** to exclude the presence of proptosis (for intraocular and intraobital causes). I will examine the anterior segment for exposure keratopathy and cockscrew vessels, check for raised intraocular pressure, and perform a dilated fundal examination for choroidal folds and intermediate uveitis. Systemically, I will check for **blood pressure, temperature,** and **neck stiffness**.

I will order a **magnetic resonance imaging of the brain and orbits with contrast and magnetic resonance venogram (disc swelling),** looking for space-occupying lesions, infective or white matter lesions, venous sinus thrombosis, and small slit-like ventricles (idiopathic intracranial hypertension + empty sella). In the absence of contraindications, I will perform a **lumbar puncture,** looking for raised opening pressure and abnormalities in cultures and biochemistry. Other investigations will include **blood tests (full blood count, erythrocyte sedimentation rate, C-reactive protein)**. If in doubt, I will perform a B scan, autofluorescence, and fundus fluorescein angiogram to differentiate from pseudopapilloedema.

> **Q** **Question 1.2 How will you Manage a Patient whose Cerebrospinal Fluid Opening Pressure is 30 mmHg, while being otherwise Normal?**

This patient is likely to have **idiopathic intracranial hypertension**. Management requires a step-wise approach and can be divided into conservative and surgical. Conservatively, I will encourage the patient to **lose weight** and **stop offending agents** (TANCOS) and refer the patient to the endocrinologist to **exclude systemic causes** (hypothyroidism, hypoparathyroidism, Cushing syndrome, or adrenal insufficiency), failing which I will start

	Bilateral Disc Swelling	Bilateral Disc Atrophy
Life threatening	Malignant hypertension, space occupying lesion raised intraocular pressure, duravenous sinus thrombosis, meningitis	Space occupying lesion
Other causes	Idiopathic intracranial hypertension, toxic/nutricient/hereditary optic neuropathy, compressive optic neuropathy, sequential optic neuritis, ischemic optic neuropathy, infiltrative optic neuropathy	Idiopathic intracranial hypertension, toxic/nutricient/hereditary optic neuropathy, space occupying lesion, sequential optic neuritis, ischemic optic neuropathy, traumatic optic neuropathy, infiltrative optic neuropathy, radiation optic neuropathy
Orbital	Thyroid eye disease, ocular ischemic syndrome, orbital tumors	Thyroid eye disease, ocular ischemic syndrome, orbital tumors
Ocular	Consecutive central retinal vein occlusion, scleritis	Retinitis pigmentosa, central retinal artery occlusion, panretinal photocoagulation
Benign causes	Pseudopapilloedema: optic disc drusen (superficial versus deep), tilted disc, myelinated nerve fibre, glial tissue, elevated disc Autofluorescence: superficial disc drusens B scan: deep disc drusens	

the patient on oral **acetazolamide** in the absence of contraindications. If that fails, I will consider second-line medications like **topiramate** (anti-epileptic) or **frusemide**. If the patient has severe headache, very high cerebrospinal fluid pressure or visual field loss, I will refer the patient to the neurosurgeon to consider **cerebrospinal fluid diversion procedures** (VP and LP shunts). If there is visual field loss without significant headache, I will consider optic nerve fenestration.

Note: Repeated therapeutic lumbar puncture to relieve cerebrospinal fluid pressure is mainly indicated in pregnant patients (not fit to undergo LP or VP shunt insertion; medications are a contraindication as well).

TANCOS

Tetracycline
Vitamin **A**
Nalidixic acid
Cyclosporin
Oral contraceptive pills
Steroid withdrawal

Note: Always exclude life-threatening causes first in patients with bilateral disc swelling.

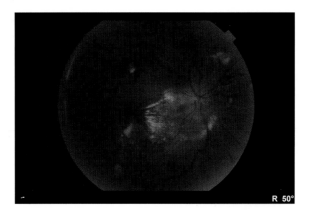

R 50°

Figure 5.2 Classical presentation of malignant hypertension with bilateral disc swelling, macula star exudation, cotton wool spots, and flame-shaped hemorrhages. The patient needs to be referred urgently to the internist for management of hypertensive emergency. Neuroretinitis could present with similar fundal features as well.

Q **Question 2 OSCE Stem: Examination showing Right Relative Afferent Pupillary Defect.**

On examination, there is **absence of anisocoria** in the light and dark. The **direct light reflex** in the right eye is **sluggish** while the left is normal; **consensual reflex** in the left eye is sluggish and normal in the right. Swinging torch tests shows a right grade 3 relative afferent pupillary defect. I will assess the **optic nerve function** by checking the visual acuity, color vision, and confrontational visual field; perform a **dilated fundal examination** for increased cup-disc ratio, pale or swollen disc, and presence of macular or retinal lesions; and check the **intraocular pressure**. I will also examine the **contiguous cranial**, test the corneal sensation (V_1) and extraocular movements (III, IV, VI) for limitation and internuclear ophthalmoplegia, and perform a **Hertel exophthalmometer** examination for proptosis.

Q **Question 3.1 Viva Stem: Patient presents Acutely with Blurring of Vision after a Punch to the Right Eye.**

Ocular trauma is a **potentially blinding condition**. I will first exclude **life-threatening injuries** and then assess for **sight-threatening injuries**. I will examine the patient's **history** for **duration since the trauma, mechanism of trauma,** whether **blurring of vision occurred acutely after trauma,** if there was any **loss of consciousness** and whether there is any **ocular pain**. I will then assess the **optic nerve function** by checking the visual acuity, relative afferent pupillary defect, color vision, and confrontational visual field; look for **proptosis** and any **lid** or **canalicular injuries**; check the **extraocular motility**; look for signs of

orbital fracture such as step deformity, crepitus, or infraorbital hypoesthesia; check the **extraocular motility;** look for signs of globe rupture or penetrating injuries, hyphema, cataract or dislocated lenses, iridodialysis, or phacodonesis; check for raised intraocular pressure, perform a **dilated fundal examination** for optic nerve swelling or surrounding hemorrhage, vitreous hemorrhage, retinal tears, detachment, or dialysis.

Note: Sight-threatening (posterior to anterior) optic canal fracture, retrobulbar hemorrhage, orbital number, optic neuropathy, choroidal rupture especially involving the macula, traumatic mac hole, retinal detachment, subluxed lens, hyphema, globe rupture/penetration/perforating injuries.

- North American Spinal Cord Injury Study (NASCIS II) showed that use of mega-dose and high-dose steroids resulted in improved neurological recovery.
- Corticosteroid Randomization After Significant Head Injury Study (CRASH) found higher mortality rates with mega-dose steroids.
- International Optic Nerve Trauma Study (IONTS) found no benefit in intravenous steroids and optic nerve canal decompression surgery.

Q **Question 3.2 Patient has Visual Acuity of "Counting Fingers with Relative Afferent Pupillary Defect on the Right and Poor Color Vision, Microscopic Hyphema, Mild Disc Swelling, and Normal Intraocular Pressure".**

This patient has **traumatic optic neuropathy** with microscopic hyphema. Traumatic optic neuropathy is an **ocular emergency**; however, treatment is **controversial**. After **excluding life-threatening** and other **sight-threatening injuries**, I will perform an **urgent computer tomography scan of the orbit** with **1-mm fine cuts looking for bony fragment compression**. If there is presence of **bony fragment compression**, the patient will require **urgent optic canal decompression** via a **transethmoidal approach**, and I will admit and co-manage the patient with the **otolaryngologist**. If there is no bone fragment, I will discuss with the patient and family members regarding the **guarded prognosis**, and the risk and benefits of **intravenous steroids**, explaining that the **benefits of steroids have not been directly proven**. If the patient presents within **eight hours**, with a **visual acuity of 6/18 or worse** in the **absence of bony compression and contraindications**, I will admit the patient and start high-dose **intravenous methylprednisolone 1 g daily in divided doses for three days followed by slow oral taper**, and monitor for improvement and side effects (dose is 250 mg qds IV x 3/7).

Note: Similar IV MP regime is also used in optic neuritis, giant cell arthritis, traumatic optic neuropathy, uveitis (VKH, SO) and TED. However, TED does not require oral taper post IV MP.

Q **Question 3.3 How many Patients can Improve after the Injury?**

Between **30% and 50%** of patients can show improvement after the acute injury.

Q **Question 3.4 What Studies do you know regarding the Treatment of Traumatic Optic Neuropathy?**

- **North American Spinal Cord Injury Study (NASCIS II)** showed that use of mega-dose and high-dose steroids resulted in improved neurological recovery.
- **Corticosteroid Randomization After Significant Head Injury (CRASH) study** found higher mortality rates with mega-dose steroids.
- **International Optic Nerve Trauma Study** found no benefit in intravenous steroids and optic nerve canal decompression surgery.

Q **Question 4.1 Viva Stem: How will you Manage a Male 70-Year-old Patient who presents with a Right-Sided Temporal Headache?**

In an elderly patient presenting with temporal headache, I will need to exclude **life-threatening** as well as **sight-threatening causes**. Life-threatening causes include **giant cell arteritis** in this age group, **space-occupying lesions** such as malignancies, and **orbital infections**. Sight-threatening causes include **orbital causes** such as thyroid eye disease, orbital inflammatory disease or orbital cellulitis, dacryoadenitis, and space-occupying lesions. **Ocular causes** include scleritis; infective keratitis; glaucoma such as angle closure, neovascular, and lens-induced; bullous keratopathy; uveitis; endophthalmitis (differentials depend on acute or chronic presentation); and optic neuritis. Other common causes include sinusitis, migraines, cluster or tension headaches, and trigeminal neuralgia.

I will examine the patient's **history** for duration of onset; if the headaches are intermittent or constant and whether they are worsening; any symptoms of raised intracranial pressure like nausea, vomiting, and tinnitus; whether the headache changes with posture; **symptoms of giant cell arteritis like tenderness of the temporal scalp, pain on combing hair, jaw claudication, and muscle pain/weakness (for polymyalgia rheumatica)**; presence of **diplopia**; any **malignancy** or **loss of weight and appetite**; and whether there is any **ocular pain, blurring of vision, halos, history of previous zoster rash**, and **migraine**.

I will first examine externally for any swellings and **prominent temporal artery**, and **palpate for tenderness and absent pulse** (occlusion). I will assess the **optic nerve function** by checking the visual acuity, relative afferent pupillary defect, color vision, and confrontational visual field, and check the optic disc for swelling or pallor. Next, I will check the **extraocular movements** looking for limitations, check the **contiguous cranial nerves** 4 and 6 as well as nerve 5 by checking the dermatomes (trigeminal neuralgia) and corneal sensation (can indicate previous zoster infection as well), check for proptosis using **Hertel's exophthalmometer**, check the **anterior segment** for uveitis, check the intraocular pressure, and examine the fundus for **vasculitis** or **retinal artery oclusion**. Systemically, I will perform an **ECG** (MI). I will check for facial tenderness and for sinusitis as well. I will investigate further by performing blood as well as radiological tests. I will take a full blood count, looking for raised white blood cell for inflammation or infection and **thrombocytosis in giant cell arteritis**, check the **erythrocyte sedimentation rate and C-reactive protein**, check the inflammatory markers like **anti-dsDNA, c and p ANCA, ANA** (GCA can be associated with autoimmune conditions), and perform imaging of the **brain and orbits**.

> **Q** **Question 4.2 How would you Manage a Patient who Defaulted and Returned Two days later with Sudden Loss of Vision (Perception of Light) and Disc Findings shown in Figure 5.3? Blood Investigations reveal Raised Thrombocytosis and Erythrocyte Sedimentation Rate of 70.**

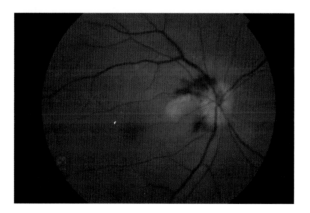

Figure 5.3 Giant cell arteritis is a devastating condition. This unfortunate patient, who was blind in the contralateral eye from an unrelated cause, presented with acute rapidly progressive loss of vision in the right eye with associated temporal headache. Final vision was hand movement in this eye.

The fundal photo of the right eye shows a **pale and diffusely swollen optic disc** with associated flame hemorrhages superiorly and inferotemporally. It is also associated with an **adjacent patch of pale edematous retina** suggestive of a **cilioretinal artery occlusion**. The rest of the fundus appears unremarkable.

In this elderly patient with **raised erythrocyte sedimentation rate, thrombocytosis,** and a **pale swollen disc,** I will be concerned about **giant cell arteritis** which is a sight- and life-threatening condition that is difficult to treat and **requires prolonged immunosuppression**. I will examine the patient's history for **fever, malaise, weight loss,** and **polymyalgia rheumatic,** as well as **pain on combing**. I will perform a **temporal artery biopsy** as soon as possible as well as a **steroid workup**. I will admit the patient and co-manage with the **rheumatologist** and **cardiologist**. I will start the patient on **intravenous high-dose methylprednisolone 1 g daily for three days in divided doses,** after which I will switch to **1 mg/kg prednisolone with prolonged treatment and slow** taper, titrate depending on the visual recovery and erythrocyte sedimentation rate levels. **Steroid treatment should not be withheld while awaiting the biopsy**. I will ideally like to perform the **biopsy within three days of commencement of steroids** up to a maximum of seven days.

Q **Question 4.3** How would you Perform a Temporal Artery Biopsy?

I will perform the procedure under informed consent in the operating theater under local anesthesia and in sterile conditions. I will **first locate the temporal artery** by palpation or ultrasound (2 cm anterior and superior to tragus), **infiltrate locally with anesthesia, incise with a Bard–Parker blade,** and **dissect down till the superficial temporal fascia** is exposed. I will identify the temporal artery, taking care not to injure the **auriculotemporal nerve, dissect the artery away from the fascia** using Weskott scissors, **ligating at two ends 3 cm apart** (at least 1.5 cm) with **4/o silk, cauterize the two ends and excise the artery,** and subsequently **close in layers with 6/o vicryl and 7/o silk for the skin**. I will start the patient on topical antibiotics and steroid ointment in the absence of contraindications.

Q **Question 4.4** What are the Complications of Temporal Artery Biopsy?

The complications are **stroke, infection, bleeding, scalp necrosis,** and **trauma to the facial nerve** and **failure to identify artery**.

Q **Question 4.5** Describe the Histopathological Specimens shown in Figures 5.4A and 5.4B.

Figure 5.4A is the **cross-sectional slide** of the artery with features of **luminal stenosis** with significant **transmural inflammation** and **fibrosis of the tunica intima**. Figure 5.4B shows the magnified view of the specimen. **Multinucleated Langerhan giant cells** are seen prominently with **loss of the internal elastic lamina**. I will examine the rest of the specimen to look for **skip lesions**. These features are consistent with **giant cell arteritis**.

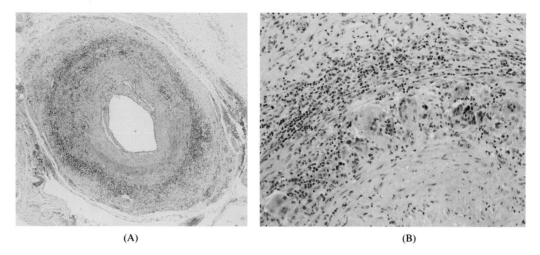

(A)   (B)

Figure 5.4 (A) Cross-section of temporal artery showing transmural inflammation and intimal fibrosis (hematoxylin and eosin stain, original magnification x20). (B) Higher magnification view of the temporal artery wall. Multinucleated giant cells are readily seen within the wall, along with an infiltrate of mixed inflammatory cells (hematoxylin and eosin stain, original magnification x200).

Histological features of giant cell arteritis:

1. Lumen occlusion
2. Loss of internal elastic lamina
3. Tunica media necrosis
4. Infiltration of inflammatory cells
5. Giant cells
6. Skipped lesions

- Giant cell arteritis is a systemic inflammatory disease affecting the medium and large-sized vessels.
- Treatment of giant cell arteritis requires slow taper 1–2 years or lifelong oral steroids.
- Titrate according to erythrocyte sedimentation rate.

Note: jaw claudication occurs as a result of masseter ischemia.

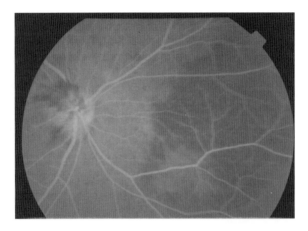

Figure 5.5 Fundus fluorescein angriography can be considered during the workup for giant cell arteritis (signs: patchy and delayed choroidal and retinal perfusion as well as possible arterial occlusion). The angiogram performed for this patient demonstrates presence of large areas of choroidal hypoperfusion nasal to the optic disc.

> **Q** **Question 5.1 Viva Stem: What are the Possible Differentials for a 30-Year-old Female who presents with Increasing Left Worse than Right Blurring of Vision?**

In this scenario, causes can be divided into life-threatening causes and sight-threatening causes. **Life-threatening causes** include malignancies like **leukemia, lymphoma, metastasis**, or **space-occupying lesions**. **Sight-threatening causes** include orbital tumors or inflammatory conditions like orbital inflammatory disease and thyroid eye disease; ocular causes such as scleritis, infective keratitis, keratoconus, glaucoma, and uveitis; and lens pathologies like subluxed lens, posterior uveitis, retinal detachments, and optic neuritis/neuropathies (differentials to offer depends on whether symptoms are acute or chronic).

> **Q** **Question 5.2 What are the Likely Causes of Pain on Ocular Movements in a Patient?**

Possible causes include **intracranial — optic neuritis, intraorbital — orbital myositis, thyroid eye disease or orbital tumors, and intraocular — scleritis.**

> **Q** **Question 5.3 Fundal Photo of the Patient.**

This is the disc photo of the patient's left eye showing a **grossly swollen hyperemic disc** with **obscuration of the blood vessels crossing the disc margin**. The vitreous appears clear and there are no choroidal folds. The macula and the rest of the retina appears normal. The patient likely has left **optic neuritis**. I will assess the optic nerve function by checking the visual acuity, relative afferent pupillary defect, and confrontational visual field, looking for anisocoria. I will check the **extraocular movements** for limitation as well as **internuclear ophthalmoplegia (multiple sclerosis)**, check for proptosis with **Hertel's exophthalmometer**, examine the **anterior segment** for uveitis, and examine the fellow eye. I will look for **systemic signs such as ataxia, hemiparesis**, or **hypoesthesia** that might suggest a demyelinating cause.

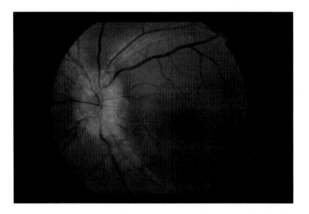

Figure 5.6   Unilateral optic disc swelling and hyperemia in a patient with left optic neuritis.

Q **Question 5.4 What are the Causes of Optic Neuritis?**

Causes of optic neuritis include **idiopathic, demyelinating** such as multiple sclerosis and neuromyelitis optica, **infective, post infectious or post vaccinations, autoimmune/ inflammatory** as well as **infiltrative**.

Infective	Non-Infection
Herpes simplex virus	Idiopathic/demyelinating
Varicella–Zoster virus	— neuromyelitis optica/multiple sclerosis
Tuberculosis	Infiltrative
Syphillis	— scarcoid
	Inflammatory
	— systemic lupus erythematosus, chronic relapsing inflammatory optic neuropathy

The Optic Neuritis Treatment Trial (ONTT) at 15 years — if ≥1 white matter lesions in MRI, risk of multiple sclerosis 72% versus 25% if there are no lesions.

Q Question 5.5 What Other Parts of the Patient's History will you Examine?

I will examine the patient's history for **duration of blurring of vision, progression,** any particular **field defect, diplopia,** and any **previous episodes of blurring of vision.** Take a **systemic history** looking for infections such as tuberculosis by asking the patient if he or she has any fever, chills, cough, night sweats, any history of sexually transmitted disease, any recent infections or sinusitis, **demyelinating conditions** such as multiple sclerosis and neuromyelitis optica by asking for **weakness and paraesthesia or loss of bowel and bladder control,** and any joint pains or rashes indicating inflammatory conditions.

Q Question 5.6 How would you Manage a Patient with Visual Acuity of 6/60 in the Left Eye and 6/12 in the Right Eye?

I will first perform **diagnostic** and **steroid workups.**

For diagnostic evaluation, I will perform a **full blood count** for raised white blood cells for infections, **erythrocyte sedimentation rate,** and **C-reactive protein,** check for infections such as **tuberculosis** by performing a **mantoux test** and **take a chest X-ray** (which can also be used for sarcoidosis hilar lymphadenopathy), do a **syphilis VDRL test** and an **aquaporin 4 antibody test,** perform a **magnetic resonance of the orbit and brain with contrast** looking for **optic nerve enhancement (T2 STIR) and wide matter lesions (T2 FLAIR),** and exclude other causes such as meningitis, space-occupying lesions, and Humphrey/Goldman visual field.

Note: Multiple sclerosis optic neuritis does not require lumbar puncture for diagnosis; offer a lumbar puncture if atypical optic neuritis is suspected

Question 5.7 Results of the MRI Scan are shown in Figures 5.7A and 5.7B.

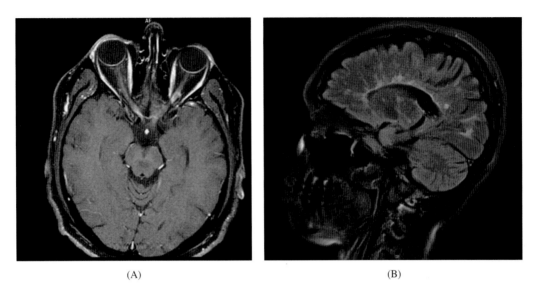

(A)   (B)

Figure 5.7 (A) Bilateral optic neuritis with enhancement of the optic nerves in this contrast fat-suppressed STIR scan. (B) Magnetic resonance imaging FLAIR scan with multiple periventricular white matter lesions with a Dawson's fingers appearance, classical for multiple sclerosis.

The left photo is the **axial cut** of the **T1-weighted magnetic resonance imaging** of the brain through the orbits with **contrast and fat suppression**. The most significant abnormalities are bilateral **hyperintense lesions at the optic nerves** that are likely enhancing, but I will compare them with non-contrasted images. The eyes are not proptosed and there are no orbital or white matter lesions noted on this cut. The right photo is the **saggital cut** of the **T2-weighted magnetic resonance imaging of the brain** using the **Fluid-Attenuated Inversion Recovery (FLAIR) sequence**. The most obvious abnormalities are the presence of multiple patches of **white matter lesions** especially in the **periventricular region** with **perpendicular projections** suggestive of Dawson's fingers. This patient has bilateral optic neuritis secondary to multiple sclerosis.

I will co-manage the patient with the neurologist. The mainstay of treatment is **systemic steroids**. I will discuss with the patient regarding the benefits and risks, explaining that intravenous steroids result in **faster resolution and better contrast, color, and visual** field, and **delay the onset of clinically definite multiple sclerosis by two years (but do not affect final visual acuity or recurrence rates)**. I will **admit** the patient and start the patient on **high-dose intravenous methylprednisolone** in the absence of contraindications **1 g per day in divided doses for three days, followed by 11 days of 1 mg/kg/day of prednisolone with fast taper**. I will monitor the patient for improvement (total 14 days of steroid treatment regime). I will also consider starting the patient on **interferone beta 1a** after discussing with the neurologist to decrease the risk of developing clinically definite multiple sclerosis.

Q Question 5.8 What are the Good Prognostic Factors for Optic Neuritis?

Good prognostic factors against development of multiple sclerosis include **absence of white matter lesions, lack of pain, presence of papillitis, peripapillary hemorrhage, macula exudates, very poor presenting visual acuity, and male gender**.

Q Question 5.9 What are the Causes of Steroid Responsive Optic Neuritis?

Causes of steroid responsive optic neuritis include **lymphoma, infiltrative** causes such as sarcoidosis and **autoimmune/inflammatory** causes associated with collagen disease.

Note: Chronic relapsing inflammatory optic neuropathy is a known cause as well.

Features of Atypical Optic Neuritis	
Symptoms	Signs
• Painless	• Severe disc hemorrhages
• Age > 50 years	• Severe disc swelling
• Bilateral simultaneous involvement	• Intracranial involvement
• Recurrent	• Uveitis
• Vision continues to worsen after two weeks	
• Vision shows no sign of improvement after five weeks	

Q Question 6.1 OSCE Stem: Examination of the Optic Disc with a DIRECT Ophthalmoscope with the following findings (see Figure 5.8). Include an Explanation of the Procedure to the Patient.

Sir, I will be examining you by shining a bright light into your right eye with this instrument. I will be coming very close to you but don't be alarmed. Please keep both eyes open and look straight ahead (at a distant fixation target). You may blink if you need to but please

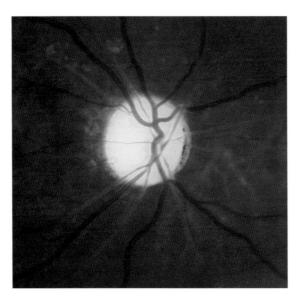

Figure 5.8   A pale optic disc in a patient with Leber's Hereditary Optic Neuropathy.

bear with me and try not to move. If it is uncomfortable, please let me know. On examination (at 60 cm), the red reflex is clear. On examination of the fundus, the disc is diffusely pale with a cup-disc ratio of 0.5 (pallor > cupping) with well-defined edges. The retinal vessels and the macula appear normal. I will complete my examination by checking the fellow eye and assessing the optic nerve function by checking the visual acuity, relative afferent papillary defect, color vision, and confrontational visual field. I will perform a full dilated fundal examination and examine the fellow eye.

Q   **Question 6.2 What are your Differentials for a Bilateral Pale Optic Disc?**

Causes of bilateral optic disc pallor can be divided into **optic neuropathy** causes and less commonly, **retinal** causes. Optic neuropathy causes include hereditary optic neuropathy; toxic, nutritional, and compressive optic neuropathy; consecutive ischaemic optic neuropathy; or consecutive optic neuritis and infiltrative lesions. It is unlikely secondary to glaucoma as there is a greater degree of pallor compared to cupping. Retinal causes include retinitis pigmentosa (less likely as arterioles are not attenuated), bilateral extensive panretinal photocoagulation, and bilateral central retinal artery occlusion (less likely as arterioles are not attenuated).

Q Question 6.3 **What are the Genes Associated with Leber's Hereditary Optic Neuropathy, what is the Prognosis, and How is it Inherited?**

The three most common genes isolated for Leber's hereditary optic neuropathy are **11778** which is the most common with the poorest prognosis, **3460**, and **14484** which is the least common of the three but has the best prognosis. It has a mitochondrial inheritance pattern.

2. Pupils

Q Question 7.1 **OSCE Stem: Examination of Elderly Patient with Bilateral Light Near Dissociation.**

On examination of this patient, there is bilateral mild **lid retraction** (collier sign) but **no abnormal head posture**. Both eyes are straight on **Hirschberg reflex**. There is **no anisocoria** in the light and in the dark. **Direct response** of the right eye is sluggish; direct response of the left eye is sluggish. **Consensual response** in the right eye is sluggish; consensual response in the left eye is sluggish. There is **no relative afferent pupillary defect**. On testing of **accommodation**, the near reflex is **brisk**. This patient has **bilateral light-near dissociation**. On examination of the extraocular movements, there is evidence of **vertical gaze palsy** and **convergence paresis**. **Vestibulo-ocular reflex** testing confirms the **supranuclear gaze palsy** (doll's eyes reflex is intact). This patient has **dorsal mid-brain syndrome**. I will look for other associated features such as **convergence spasm, accommodation paresis**, or **spasm**, check for **convergence retraction nystagmus** using an optokinetic nystagmus drum (rotate downwards), and check for **skew deviation** (Wong's upright-supine test). The likely etiology is **stroke, tumor**, or **Wernicke's encephalopathy in this age group**. Other differentials to light-near dissociation include Argyll Robertson pupils and bilateral tonic pupils. I will perform **neuroimaging** to localize the lesion.

Note: Do offer vestibulo-ocular reflex (doll's eyes reflex) check after checking for limitation of supraductions and infraductions.

Q Question 7.2 **What are the Differentials to Bilateral Vertical Gaze Palsy?**

Differentials include **dorsal mid-brain syndrome with supranuclear gaze palsy, progressive supranuclear gaze palsy, myasthenia, thyroid eye disease, bilateral orbital wall fractures, congenital fibrosis of the extraocular muscles** (versus Mobius = horizontal), and **early chronic progressive external ophthalmoplegia**.

Q Question 8 OSCE Stem: Examination of Tonic Pupil.

On examination of this patient, there is **no abnormal head posture** and **no ptosis**, and eyes appear **straight on Hirschberg light reflex on primary gaze**. In the **light**, there is **anisocoria** with the right pupil larger than the left. On examination in the **dark**, there is **reduced anisocoria** with the right slightly larger than the left. The abnormal pupil is on the right. On checking **direct light reflex**, the **right eye is sluggish** and the left eye is brisk. On checking **consensual reflex**, the consensual reflex **in the right eye is sluggish** and in the left eye is brisk. There is **no relative afferent pupillary defect by the reverse method**. In the light, the **near reflex is sluggish in the right eye but faster than the light reflex**, indicating **light-near dissociation**. This patient has a right **tonic pupil**. I will complete my examination by checking under the slit lamp for **vermiform movements**. I will perform a **pilocarpine 0.125% test** (reversal of anisocoria secondary to denervation hypersensitivity) and check for **tendon areflexia** (Holmes–Adie syndrome). The patient is likely to have a right tonic pupil. Other causes of a tonic pupil include diabetes, syphilis, trauma and degeneration and familial dysautonomia syndrome. Other differentials to light-near dissociation include dorsal mid-brain syndrome.

Note: Tests to differentiate the different causes of large pupil: 0.125% for Adie's pupil, 1% for CN III palsy, 4% for pharmacologically dilated pupil.

Tonic Pupil (Vermiform Movements of Iris or Sectorial Palsy)		
Primary	**Secondary**	**Site**
• Adie's syndrome • Holmes–Adie syndrome (areflexia)	• DM • Syphilis • Trauma • Degeneration • PD • PSP • Iatrogenic • Tumor • Myotonia dystrophica • Dysautonomia (e.g. Riley–Day syndrome)	• Ciliary ganglion • Short ciliary nerves

Q Question 9.1 OSCE Stem: Examination of Horner's Pupil.

On general examination, there is **partial** right ptosis obscuring the visual axis with associated **inverse ptosis** of the lower lid. Both eyes are straight on **Hirschberg reflex**. In the **light**, there is **mild anisocoria** with the right pupil **smaller** than the left. In the **dark**, there is **increased** anisocoria with the right pupil smaller than the left. Direct light reflexes and

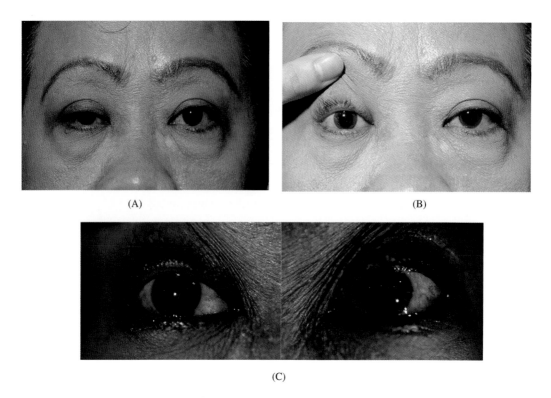

(A)

(B)

(C)

Figures 5.9A–5.9C This sequence of photos illustrates the characteristic features in a patient with right Horner's syndrome. The right lid is partially ptotic. In the light, there is anisocoria with the right pupil being smaller than the left that is worsened in the dark.

consensual reflexes are normal. There is no relative afferent pupillary defect. I will check for other features of Horner's syndrome: I will palpate for **anhidrosis, iris heterochromia, and hypotony**; assess the optic nerve function (orbital apex); perform a dilated fundal examination looking for optic disc swelling or pallor; assess the extraocular motility, corneal sensation, hearing, and facial nerve function; and check for long tract signs (sensory/motor/cerebella — lateral medullary syndrome). I will examine for **etiology**, looking for nail clubbing and thenar wasting, and auscultate the apex of the lung (Pancoast tumor) for cervical scars (carotid dissection) as well as neck masses. I will perform **pharmacological tests to confirm the diagnosis and localize the lesion**. I will administer **cocaine** 10% or **apraclonidine** 0.5% to confirm Horner's syndrome and **hydroxyamphetemine** 1% or **phenylephrine** 1% to determine the level of the lesion.

Q Question 9.2 What are Some Syndromes associated with Horner's Syndrome?

Syndromes include Foville (Cranial nerves 5, 6, 7, 8, Horner's) and lateral medullary syndrome (Cranial nerve 5 [with ipsilateral face and contralateral body nociception and temperature sensation loss], 9, 10, cerebellar).

> Dangerous Horner's syndrome
> 1. Neck pain — carotid dissection
> 2. Lung cancer — Pancoast tumor
> 3. Neuroblastoma — in children (a/w opsoclonus and Racoon's eye)
> Management: MRI + MRA orbits, head and neck with contrast + CT thorax

Q Question 9.3 How do you Differentiate Pre-Ganglionic from Post-Ganglionic Horner's Syndrome Clinically? What is the Reason?

I can check for **anhidrosis** of the ipsilateral face as the **sudomotor fibers** follow the external carotid artery. Sweating will be intact in third-order lesions.

3. Visual Fields

Q Question 10.1 OSCE Stem: Visual Field Examination of a Patient with a Representative Humphrey Visual Field Test Result shown in Figures 5.10A and 5.10B.

On examination, this patient has left-sided superior homonymous quadrantinopia. The lesion is right **retrochiasmal** (optic tract to optic radiations to occipital). I will check the visual acuity; look for **long tract signs** and **temporal lobe signs** such as auditory hallucinations; examine the patient's history for epilepsy, formed visual hallucinations, and occipital lobe symptoms such as unformed visual hallucinations; and perform a **Humphrey visual field test** for congruity. In summary, this patient has a left-sided superior homonymous quadrantinopia secondary to a right retrochiasmal lesion. I will also perform **neuroimaging tests** to confirm the diagnosis.

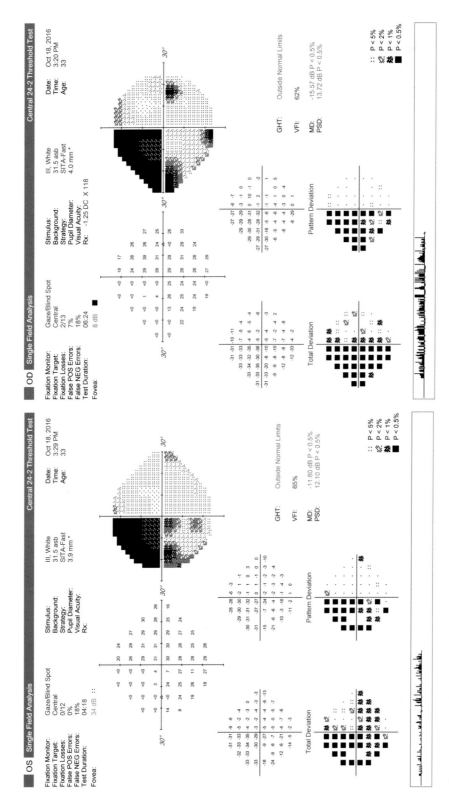

Figures 5.10A and 5.10B These are the representative Humphrey visual field test results in a patient with right temporal lobe space occupying lesion with an associated left superior quadrantinopia.

Q Question 10.2 If the Visual Field Defect is Inferior, what Signs would you Look Out for?

If the visual field defect is inferior, the lesion is likely in the **parietal** lobe or **occipital** lobe. I will look for **dominant lobe signs** such as acalculia agraphia agnosia and left–right disorientation, as well as **non-dominant lobe signs** such as dyscalculia, hemineglect, and constructional apraxia. I will also look for **pursuit deficit** (frontal lobes control contralateral saccades and parietal lobes control ipsilateral pursuits) and check for **asymmetric response with the optokinetic nystagmus drum (unable to pursuit to ipsilateral side)**. Occipital **lobe lesions** will have normal pursuit and symmetrical optokinetic nystagmus response.

Q Question 10.3 What are the Causes in a Young Patient.

The causes in a young patient include **space-occupying lesion, demyelinating disease such as multiple sclerosis**, and **trauma**, as well as **arteriovenous malformations**.

Note: If it is quadrantopia, there is no need to check optic nerve function as it is posterior to the lateral geniculate ganglion, so there will be no relative afferent pupillary defect or optic disc pallor. Temporal lobe features include déjà vu epilepsy, uncinate epilepsy, aphasia, and formed visual hallucinations.

Q Question 11.1 OSCE Stem: Visual Field Examination of a Patient with a Representative Humphrey Visual Field Test shown in Figures 5.11A and 5.11B.

On examination, this patient has bitemporal hemianopia. It is likely secondary to a **chiasmal lesion** such as a pituitary adenoma. I will assess the optic nerve function by checking the visual acuity, relative afferent pupillary defect, color vision, and red cap perimetry; perform a dilated fundal examination for **bow tie optic disc atrophy** or optic disc pallor; assess the **contiguous cranial nerves** such as the third, fourth, and sixth nerve on extraocular movements, as well as corneal sensation for the fifth nerve that might suggest **cavernous sinus involvement**. I will check for **post-fixational blindness** and **see-saw nystagmus,** and examine the patient's history for **hemifield slip** and **visual hallucinations**. I will examine **systemically for acromegaly and Cushing's syndrome**; examine the patient's history for growth spurt, **galactorrhea**, infertility, and obesity, as well as any **previous trauma surgery radiation** or **malignancies**; and perform a **Goldman visual field test** and **neuroimaging** to confirm the diagnosis.

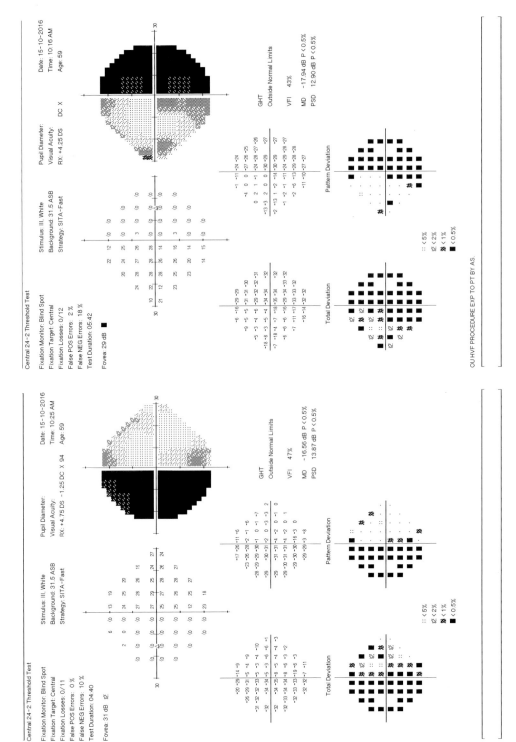

Figures 5.11A and 5.11B These are the representative Humphrey visual field test results in a patient with a large pituitary macroadenoma causing a bitemporal hemianopia.

Q Question 11.2 What are the Causes of Bitemporal Hemianopia?

Bitemporal hemianopia is secondary to a **chiasmal lesion** which is most commonly due to a **pituitary adenoma**. Other causes include **benign tumors** such as meningioma, glioma, **craniopharyngioma, Rathke pouch cyst**, fibrous dysplasia, and subarachnoid cyst, as well as **malignancies** such as metastasis and nasopharyngeal carcinoma. Other causes include **demyelinating conditions** such as multiple sclerosis and **inflammatory conditions** like Tolosa–Hunt syndrome, **post-trauma** or **surgery**, and **post-radiotherapy**.

Q Question 11.3 What are the Differentials to a Chiasmal Lesion?

Other causes of bitemporal hemianopia include **bilateral nasal sectoral retinitis pigmentosa, bilateral nasal retinal schisis or detachment, tilted optic disc, bilateral dermatochalasis, bilateral optic disc coloboma**, and **ethambutol toxicity**.

Note: binasal visual field defect = empty sella syndrome (associated with idiopathic intracranial hypertension) or bilateral internal carotid aneurysm.

Q Question 11.4 How would you Investigate this Patient.

Investigation can be divided into **ocular** and **systemic**. Systemically, I will co-manage the patient with the **endocrinologist** and **neurosurgeon**, perform a **magnetic resonance imaging of the brain** and **pituitary with contrast**, and check for **hormonal dysfunction** such as **prolactin levels, growth hormone**, and **cortisol levels**. Ocular investigations will include monitoring with formal visual field perimetry as well as **optical coherence tomography** for prognostication.

Q Question 11.5 Describe the Scan shown in Figure 5.12.

This is the coronal cut of a T1-weighted magnetic resonance imaging of the brain through the pituitary with contrast. The most obvious abnormality is a large well-defined hyperintense homogenous mass arising from the suprasellar region with mass effect, compressing upward on the optic chiasm (white arrow) but it is not invading the adjacent cavernous sinus. I will compare it with the T1-weighted non-contrasted scan but the lesion is likely to be enhancing. The ventricles are not dilated. This is likely a pituitary macroadenoma.

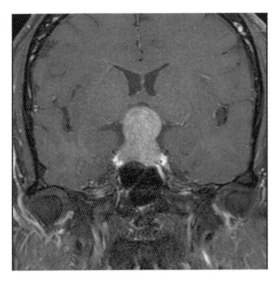

Figure 5.12   Pituitary macroadenoma compressing the optic chiasm.

Q   **Question 11.6 How would you Manage this Patient?**

I will co-manage the patient with the **endocrinologist** and **neurosurgeon**. If It is a **prolactinoma**, I will start the patient on **dopamine agonist** like **bromocriptine** or **cabergoline** in the absence of contraindications. If it is causing significant compression on the chiasm with visual field defects, I will consider **transsphenoidal hypophysectomy** if the patient is fit. If the patient is not fit for surgery, then **radiotherapy/gamma knife** can be considered.

Figures 5.13A and 5.13B show another visual field defect commonly tested during exams.

Q   **Question 12 OSCE Stem: Visual Field Examination of a Patient with the Representative Humphrey Visual Field Test shown in Figure 5.14.**

On examination, this patient has **left inferior altitudinal defect**. I will assess the **optic nerve function** by checking the visual acuity, relative afferent pupillary defect, color vision, and red cap perimetry; check the **contiguous cranial nerves**, assessing for **proptosis using Hertel's exophthalmometer**; check the **intraocular pressure**; perform a **dilated fundal examination** for **optic disc pallor, swelling**, or **increased cup-disc ratio or disc at risk**; and look for **retinal pathologies** such as superior retinal detachments, superior retinoschisis, superior retinitis pigmentosa (asymmetrical retinitis pigmentosa in monocular; if bilateral then consider symmetrical retinitis pigmentosa), superior branch retinal artery, or vein occlusion (especially with superior panretinal photocoagulation). I will examine

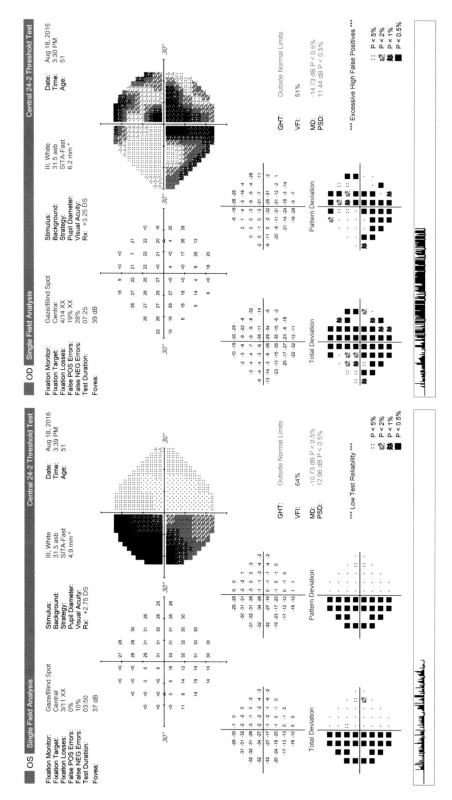

Figures 5.13A and 5.13B Right junctional scotoma — right central scotoma with left temporal visual field defect.

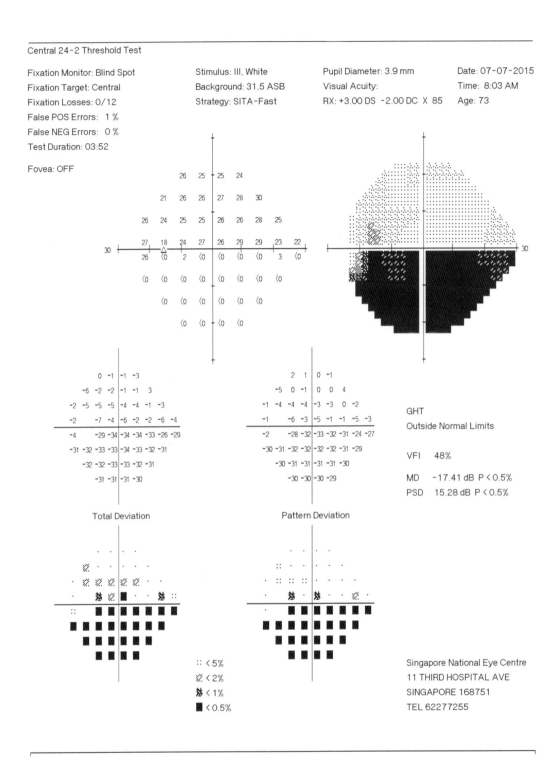

Central 24-2 Threshold Test

Fixation Monitor: Blind Spot
Fixation Target: Central
Fixation Losses: 0/12
False POS Errors: 1 %
False NEG Errors: 0 %
Test Duration: 03:52

Fovea: OFF

Stimulus: III, White
Background: 31.5 ASB
Strategy: SITA-Fast

Pupil Diameter: 3.9 mm
Visual Acuity:
RX: +3.00 DS -2.00 DC X 85

Date: 07-07-2015
Time: 8:03 AM
Age: 73

Total Deviation

Pattern Deviation

GHT
Outside Normal Limits

VFI   48%

MD   -17.41 dB P < 0.5%
PSD   15.28 dB P < 0.5%

:: < 5%
⚹ < 2%
⊛ < 1%
■ < 0.5%

Singapore National Eye Centre
11 THIRD HOSPITAL AVE
SINGAPORE 168751
TEL 62277255

Figure 5.14 This patient presented with loss of inferior visual field when he woke up. The Humphrey visual field results show a characteristic inferior altitudinal field defect respecting the horizontal meridian.

the patient's history for vascular risk factors; obstructive sleep apnea or use of nocturnal hypotensives; presence of temporal headache, jaw claudication, malaise, or loss of weight, as well as previous trauma or recurrent optic neuritis. Differentials will include **optic neuritis, compressive optic neuropathy, anterior ischaemic optic neuropathy**, and **glaucoma**, as well as retinal causes such as **superior retinal detachment, superior retinitis pigmentosa, branch retinal artery**, or **vein occlusion**.

Q Question 13 OSCE Stem: Visual Field Examination of a Patient with Representative Humphrey Visual Field Test Results shown in Figures 5.15A and 5.15B.

On examination, the patient has bilateral centrocecal scotoma likely secondary to bilateral **optic neuropathy** (macular lesions are more likely for central scotomas). I will check the visual acuity, relative afferent pupillary defect, color vision, and red cap perimetry, and perform a dilated fundal examination for **optic disc pallor** or **disc swelling**. Optic neuropathy causes include hereditary optic neuropathy, nutritional or toxic neuropathy, consecutive optic neuritis, space-occupying lesions bilaterally, infiltrative, bilateral traumatic or post radiation neuropathy. I will perform a Humphrey visual field test for assessment of the scotoma.

VFD	Enlarged Blind Spot	Centrocecal	Altitudinal	Central/ Paracentral	Arcuate	Bitemporal
Nerve	• Papilloedema • Optic disc drusen • Coloboma • PPA • Optic neuritis	• Hereditary • Toxic • Nutritional • Optic neuritis • Compressive • NTG	• Ischemic • Compressive • Optic neuritis	• Hereditary • Toxic • Nutritional • Optic neuritis • Compressive • NTG	Glaucoma Optic neuritis Compressive	• Chiasmal lesions • ON coloboma
Retinal	• MEWDS • Idiopathic enlarged blind spot syndrome		• HRAO • HRVO • RD • retinitis pigmentosa • Retinoschisis		• branch retinal artery occlusion • branch retinal vein occlusion • Retinal coloboma	• Binasal RP • Binasal retinoschisis
Macula				• Mac hole • Mac scar • Mac branch RAO/RVO • CSCR • AMD		
Others						• Bilateral dermatochlasis

Note: Constricted VF late staged papilledema, glaucoma, retinitis pigmentosa, PRP. macula sparing visual field defect suggests an occipital lobe lesion due to dual supply from MCA (infarct) and PCA (supply tip of occipital calcarine fissure).

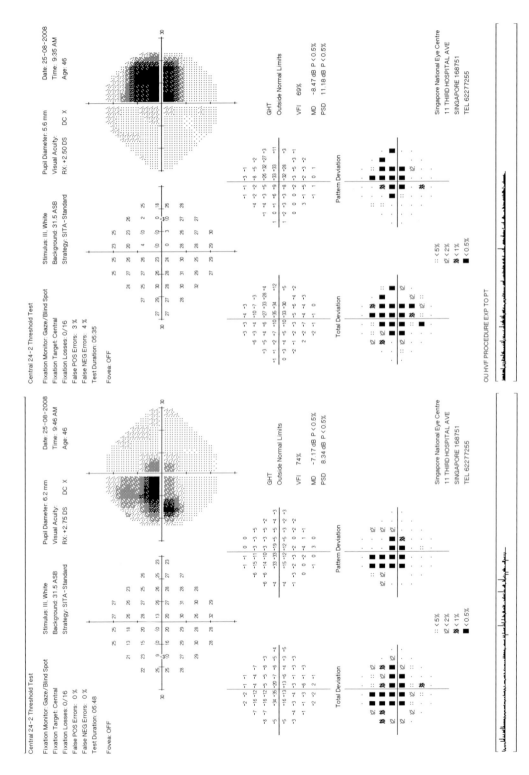

Figures 5.15A and 5.15B This patient presented with progressive bilateral blurring of vision. On further questioning, it was found that he had tuberculosis and was treated with ethambutol. He developed toxic optic neuropathy with bilateral centrocecal scotoma.

4. Ptosis and Ocular Motility

Q **Question 14.1 Viva Stem: How would you Manage Patient who Presents with Partial Ptosis and Diplopia?**

I will examine the patient's history for duration of onset, whether it is **progressive, binocular, or monocular** diplopia, **vertical, horizontal**, or **oblique**; any recent head injury, nausea, or vomiting; systemic vascular risk factors; presence of **variability** or **features of generalized myasthenia** such as fatiguability; diurnal variation; proximal myopathy; and dysphonia. I will examine the patient and perform the **Hirschberg** test in primary gaze to look ocular deviation, check the pupils for **anisocoria**, and assess the **optic nerve function** by checking the visual acuity, relative afferent pupillary defect, confrontational visual field, and color vision. I will check the **extraocular movement**, looking for limitations as well as features of **aberrant regeneration** (do not say if the stem is an acute presentation) and check for **features of myasthenia** such as weak orbicularis; lash sign; peak sign; Cogan lid twitch; and fatigability. I will check the **contiguous cranial nerves**, especially the fourth nerve, corneal sensation and sixth nerve palsy, perform a **dilated fundal examination** for disc swelling, check for proptosis using a **Hertel's exophthalmometer** (suggestive of orbital apex syndrome), and check for **long tract signs**. I will assess the ptosis, checking for deep superior sulcus and lid retraction on downgaze, and measure for palpebral aperture, marginal reflex distance, levator function, lid crease height, Bell's phenomenon, and lagophthalmos.

Q **Question 14.2 This Patient's Pupils are Normal, there is No Fatigability, but there are Limitations in Adduction Depression and Elevation.**

This patient has **partial third nerve palsy sparing the pupils**. The main aim is to **exclude life-threatening space-occupying lesions** such as a **posterior communicating cerebral artery aneurysm**. If the patient is non-compliant to follow-up, I will admit the patient for urgent **computer tomography brain scan and angiogram with contrast**, or **magnetic resonance imaging of the brain and angiogram with contrast**. If the patient is compliant to follow-up, I will monitor the patient closely and **review daily for a week to look for evolvement**.

Q **Question 14.3 How would you Manage a Patient whose Magnetic Resonance Angiography Results show a Posterior Communicating Artery Aneurysm?**

Posterior communicating artery aneurysm is a life-threatening condition. I will urgently refer the patient to the radiologist for **endovascular coiling**. If that fails, I will refer the patient to the neurosurgeon for **surgical clipping**.

- Computer tomography with angiography can pick up smaller aneurysms than a magnetic resonance angiography can.
- Gold standard: Four-vessel angiogram with digital subtraction.

Patients presenting acutely that do not require a scan include elderly patients with known vascular risk factors and patients with complete ptosis with pupil sparing and no features of aberrant regeneration.

Q Question 14.4 How would you Investigate a Patient who has Features of Fatigability?

I will perform tests in the clinic including **ice pack test** looking for improvement of ptosis by at least **2 mm after 2 min or Tensilon test** (endrophonium HCL) or **neostigmine test**. I will perform a blood test for **anti-acetylcholine receptor antibodies** and a **thyroid function test**, order a **repetitive nerve stimulation test** looking for **decremental response** and a **single-fiber electromyogram** looking for **jitters** and **variability**. I will perform a **computer tomography scan of the chest** to look for presence of **thymoma**. If the blood tests are negative, I can consider checking for **anti-skeletal muscle antibodies** and **anti-muscle specific kinase (SMA, MSK)**.

Q Question 14.5 Ice Pack Test Results.

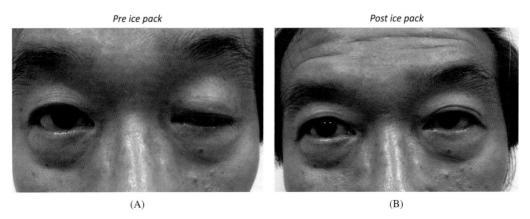

Pre ice pack — (A) *Post ice pack* — (B)

Figures 5.16A and 5.16B Positive ice pack test for ocular myasthenia gravis.

This is the partial facial photo of the patient. The left photo shows left more than right partial ptosis with the left **obscuring the visual axis**. The eyes appear grossly central on straight gaze. Post-ice pack test there is **improvement of bilateral ptosis**, more marked on the left. I will measure the extent on improvement but it is likely more than 2 mm on the left. This is a **positive** ice pack test suggestive of **ocular myasthenia gravis**.

Q Question 14.6 How would you Manage?

Management can be divided into **systemic** and **ocular**. If there are features of **generalized myasthenia**, I will co-manage the patient with a **neurologist** and admit and start the patient on **immunouppressants** in the absence of contraindications (KIV IVIG and plasmapheresis). This patient has ptosis as well as diplopia; hence I will start the patient on **pyridostigmine** with **propantheline** cover as well as **oral steroids**. (Legacy treatment: Admit the patient for monitoring during the initiation of oral steroids due to the risk of myasthenic crisis.) Other measures to alleviate his ocular symptoms include **lid crutches**, **Bangerter foil**, and **Fresnel prisms**.

Q Question 14.7 How do you Perform a Tensilon Test?

The Tensilon test is a diagnostic test for thyroid eye disease with **80% sensitivity**. I will perform the test under informed consent in the treatment room with **constant cardiac monitoring** with **resuscitation trolley** and **0.6 mg atropine on standby**. I will inform patient of the possible side effects such as **life-threatening complications** like **bradycardia hypotension**, and **bronchospasm**, as well as **common side effects** like **sweating**, **salivation**, and **nausea colic (SLUDGE)**. I will dilute **10 mg of endrophonium hydrochloride in 10 mL of normal saline**, injecting intravenously **2 mL**, watching for **improvement of ptosis** and **extraocular movements** over **2 min**, failing which I will inject another 2 mL and watch for 2 min for improvement. If there is still no response, I will then inject the **remaining 6 mL** and watch for improvement.

Note: Endrophonium hydrochloride is an anti-acetylcholinesterase inhibitor.

	Tensilon (Endrophonium Hydrochloride)	Neostigmine
Route	Intravenous (IV)	Intramuscular (IM)
Dose	10 mg in 10 mL	0.02–0.04 mg/kg (Asian — 1.5 mg)
Atropine	0.6 mg IV on standby	0.6 mg IM given together
Duration	2 min	30 min
Outcome measurement	Ptosis, EOM	Ptosis, EOM, Prism Cover Test, HESS

SLUDGE

Salivation: stimulation of the salivary glands
Lacrimation: stimulation of the lacrimal glands (tearing)
Urination: relaxation of the internal sphincter muscle of urethra, and contraction of the detrusor muscles
Diaphoresis: stimulation of the sweat glands
Gastrointestinal upset: smooth muscle tone changes causing gastrointestinal problems, including diarrhea
Emesis: Vomiting

Q **Question 15.1 OSCE Stem: Examine the Patient's Extraocular Movements depicted in Figures 5.17A–5.17I.**

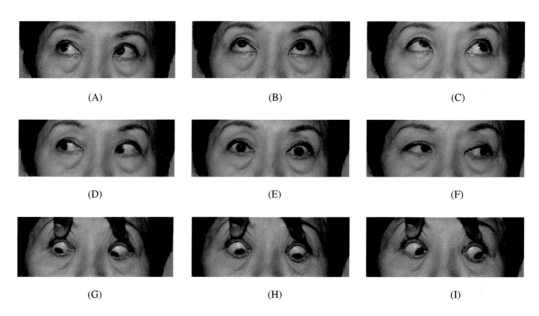

(A) (B) (C)

(D) (E) (F)

(G) (H) (I)

Figures 5.17A–5.17I This patient presented with acute vertical diplopia. Note the presence of hypertropia on primary gaze as well as over elevation on adduction. She was subsequently diagnosed with right superior oblique palsy with good spontaneous recovery.

On examination of the patient, she has a left **face turn** and **head tilt chin down position**. On **correction of the abnormal head posture**, there is a **right-over-left** hypertropia on Hirschberg light reflex. There is **over elevation on adduction of the right eye, with associated inferior oblique overaction on levoelevation and superior oblique underaction on levodepression**. This is confirmed on **testing ductions**. I will perform a **cover–uncover and alternate cover test with and without glasses for near and distance vision with prisms**. The alternate cover test confirms a right-over-left hypertropia. I will perform the **Parks 3 step test**. On right face turn (left gaze), right-over-left hypertropia is accentuated. On left face turn (right gaze), the hypertropia is reduced. On right head tilt, the hypertropia is increased. On left head tilt, the hypertropia is reduced. In summary, this patient has a right-over-left hypertropia secondary to **right fourth nerve palsy**. Differentials include **skew deviation (incyclotorsion)** and **myasthenia gravis**. I will examine the patient's history for **vascular risk factor** and **head injury, perform a family album tomography scan, check the vertical fusion range** (normal 3–5), **perform a double Maddox rod** (excyclotorsion), **perform a dilated fundal examination for excyclotorsion**, and **check optic nerve function** and **contiguous cranial nerves**.

1. Purpose of excyclotorsion assessment:
   If > 10 degrees → likely bilateral CN IV →associated with a chin down posture
   If absent excyclotorsion → possibly congenital
   If incyclotorsion is present → possibly skew deviation (WUST)
2. Other differentials include IO overaction with ET/XT that was previously operated on
3. Normal vertical fusion range between 3–5 prism diopters
4. Always offer to check extraocular motility after cover/uncover tests

Note: Dissociated vertical deviation vs CN4 vs Skew deviation
Dissociated vertical deviation: abduction, elevation, excyclotorsion

CN4 palsy: excyclotorsion and adduction

Skew: incyclotorsion, hypertropia (WUST test (upright/supine test): hypertropia deviation reduced on lying supine).

Q **Question 15.2 What are the Causes of Vertical Squints?**

Differentials include **thyroid eye disease, myasthenia, orbital wall fracture, fourth nerve and third nerve palsy, Brown's syndrome (V), and inferior oblique palsy (A),** as well as **dissociated vertical deviation, double elevator palsy, and congenital fibrosis.**

There are several ways to differentiate dissociated vertical deviation from hypertropia. Firstly, dissociated vertical deviation occurs in **all positions of upgaze** while hypertropia from fourth nerve palsy in the left eye occurs in right elevation. In dissociated vertical deviation, there will be **no corresponding hypotropia** of the right eye as compared to left fourth nerve palsy. Thirdly, **only a base-down prism in the left eye** will correct the ocular deviation from dissociated vertical deviation while either a base-up prism in the right eye or base-down prism in the left eye can correct the misalignment in left fourth nerve palsy. Correction of the dissociated vertical deviation during cover–uncover test is slow compared to fourth nerve palsy which is rapid. Dissociated vertical deviation is associated with excyclotorsion and abduction while superior oblique palsy is associated with excyclotorsion and adduction.

Q **Question 16** OSCE Stem: EOM Examination for Brown's Syndrome.

On examination of this patient, there is limited elevation of the right eye in upgaze and in levoelevation. Duction confirms presence of **supraduction deficit in elevation and levoelevation** which is associated with **a V pattern on vertical gaze**. I will perform a **cover–uncover and alternate cover test with and without glasses for near and distance vision with prisms**, perform a **forced duction test**, examine the patient's **history for trauma, recent infections**, and **ocular surgeries**. I will check the **contiguous cranial nerves**; assess the optic nerve function by checking the visual acuity, relative afferent pupillary defect, color vision, and confrontational visual fields; perform a dilated fundal examination for optic disc swelling or pallor; check the anterior segment for surgery scars; and perform a **family album tomography scan** for **abnormal head posture**. This patient is likely to have Brown's syndrome. Differentials include **inferior oblique palsy** and **myasthenia**.

Q **Question 17.1** OSCE Stem: Examine the Patient's Extraocular Movements as depicted in Figures 5.18A–5.18I.

On examination of the patient, he has left partial ptosis obscuring the visual axis. On lifting the lids, the left eye was seen to **deviate outward** with the **Hirschberg light reflex** in primary gaze. There is **limitation of left eye movement in all gazes** apart from lateral gaze confirmed on testing of ductions as well. There are **no abnormal lid movements** (for

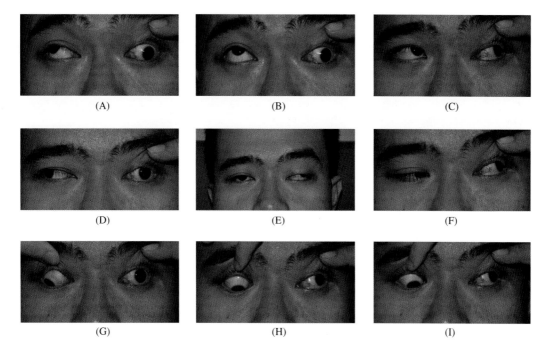

(A)	(B)	(C)
(D)	(E)	(F)
(G)	(H)	(I)

Figures 5.18A–5.18I This patient presents to the Accident and Emergency department complaining of acute diplopia with left partial ptosis. It is critical to assess for pupil involvement to exclude a life-threatening space-occupying lesion.

aberrant regeneration) on right gaze or downgaze. **Intorsion** is intact on testing in left gaze and downgaze. Convergence is non-binocular. I will **check the pupils** for anisocoria that is worse in the light and features of **aberrant regeneration**, contiguous cranial nerves, and optic nerve function such as visual acuity, relative afferent pupillary defect by reverse method to see if there is anisocoria, color vision, confrontational visual field, and direct visualization of the optic nerve. I will examine the patient's history for headache, trauma, and vascular risk factors.

> **Q** **Question 17.2 Examination reveals Anisocoria with Left Greater than Right and Worse in the Light.**

This patient has partial third nerve palsy with pupil involvement. I would be worried about a space-occupying lesion such as a posterior communicating artery aneurysm. I will order an urgent computer tomography scan of the brain with angiogram (or magnetic resonance imaging of the brain with contrast and magnetic resonance angiography).

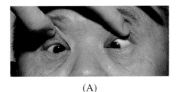 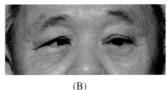 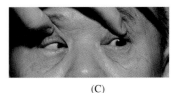

(A)   (B)   (C)

Figures 5.19A–5.19C   Right sixth nerve palsy.

On examination of the patient, it was found that the patient has a **right face turn**. On straightening of the head, the right eye is **deviated inwards** with the **Hirschberg light reflex** in primary gaze. On left gaze, eye movements are full with no abnormal lid movements. On right gaze, there is **limitation in the right eye**. On testing ductions, there is confirmed presence of **abduction deficit** in the right eye. Vertical movements are normal. Convergence is intact/binocular. This patient has a right abduction deficit likely secondary to a **right sixth nerve palsy**. Differentials include myasthenia gravis, medial orbital fracture, thyroid eye disease, Duane's syndrome, longstanding congenital esotropia, and convergence spasm. I will assess the optic nerve function by checking the visual acuity, relative afferent papillary defect, color vision, and confrontational visual field, and check the **optic disc for swelling** (false localizing sign). I will assess the lids for fatigability (myasthenia), check for proptosis with Hertel's exophthalmometer, assess the contiguous cranial nerves, check for long tract signs (and refer the patient to an ENT specialist to screen for nasopharyngeal cancer in South Asians) and examine the patient's history for vascular risk factors.

Q   **Question 18.2 How would you Manage this Patient.**

I will examine the patient's history for **onset** and **duration**, whether it is **acute** or **progressive**, any presence of **vascular risk factors**, any **ear blockage** or **tinnitus** (for nasopharyngeal carcinoma), variability to exclude **myasthenia gravis**, any blurring of vision, any headache, nausea, vomiting, and tinnitus that vary with posture (for **raised intracranial pressure**), and any **trauma** or **malignancy**. If the patient has progressive worsening, symptoms, or signs of raised intracranial pressures (such as papilloedema), history of malignancy, or lack of vascular risk factors, I will perform a **magnetic resonance imaging of the brain and orbit with contrast with venogram**. In the meantime, I will refer the patient to the otolaryngologist to exclude nasopharyngeal carcinoma.

Management can be divided into **systemic** and **ocular**. Systemically, I will co-manage the patient with the internist to treat the underlying cause. Initial ocular management will be to **alleviate symptoms of diplopia** such as applying prisms, Bangerter foil, patching, and botulinum injection into the medial rectus. Surgical intervention is considered in patients with persistent diplopia. If there is acceptable residual lateral rectus function, combined medial rectus recession with lateral rectus resection can be considered. If there is poor residual function, muscle sharing procedures such as Jensen's or Hummelsheim's procedures can be considered.

(An alternative question would be: When would you perform neuroimaging in patients with sixth cranial nerve palsy? Answer: When the patient is young; when there is an absence of ischemic risk factors; when there is progressive, non-isolated sixth cranial nerve palsy and a lack of spontaneous recovery; and when there is a history of malignancy and signs and symptoms of raised intracranial pressure.)

> **Q** **Question 19 OSCE Stem: Examine the Patient's Extraocular Movements as depicted in Figures 5.20A–5.20C.**

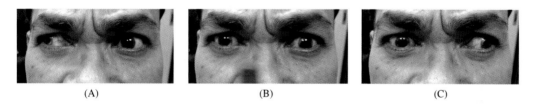

(A)   (B)   (C)

Figures 5.20A–5.20C This patient had bilateral internuclear ophthalmoplegia secondary to multiple sclerosis. Ocular myasthenia might mimic the presence of an internuclear ophthalmoplegia as well.

On examination of the patient, there is no abnormal head posture and eyes are straight on **Hirschberg light reflex** in primary gaze. On right gaze, there is **limitation of the left eye** with an **abducting nystagmus** in the right eye. Testing of **ductions** confirms an adduction deficit in the left eye. On left gaze, there is **limitation of the right eye** with an **abducting nystagmus in the left eye**. Testing of ductions confirms an adduction deficit in the right eye. Vertical gazes and convergence are intact. This patient has **bilateral internuclear ophthalmoplegia**. My differential is ocular myasthenia. I will check the optic nerve function (for optic neuritis secondary to multiple sclerosis) such as visual acuity, relative afferent pupillary defect, color vision, and confrontational visual field, and direct visualization of the optic nerve for pallor or swelling. I will assess for fatigability and for long track signs (especially cerebellar signs for multiple sclerosis).

5. Nystagmus

Q Question 20 OSCE Stem: Examination of Patient with Face Turn and Congenital Nystagmus.

On examination, the patient has a right face turn. On straightening of the head, there is **binocular pendular conjugate horizontal nystagmus** on primary gaze. There is **no titubation**. On covering of each eye, there is increased nystagmus of the uncovered eye suggestive of **latent nystagmus**. On right gaze, eye movements are full and there is pendular horizontal nystagmus. On left gaze, eye movements are full, and nystagmus is horizontal but **dampened** suggestive of a **null point**. On upgaze and downgaze, movements are full and nystagmus **remains horizontal**. Therefore, nystagmus is **uniplanar**. On **convergence**, nystagmus is dampened. This patient has features of congenital nystagmus.

I will examine the patient's history for **onset** (birth or two to three months after birth), **absence of oscillopsia, reduction during rest and convergence, and worst on fixation**; checking for **paradoxical optokinetic nystagmus drum response** (fast pursuit, slow saccades; on turning toward the patient's right, there is presence of fast pursuit to the right and slow saccades to the left, suggestive of paradoxical optokinetic nystagmus response); check the **visual acuity binocularly** and **monocularly with fogging for both near and distance vision with and without AHP correction (on occlusion, latent nystagmus will worsen the visual acuity)**; and check for **refraction** and **stereopsis**. I will also examine the **anterior** and **posterior segment** for features such as **ocular albinism, aniridia**, and **foveal and optic nerve hypoplasia**.

Q Question 21 OSCE Stem: Examination of Downbeat Nystagmus.

On examination, this patient has downbeat nystagmus **worse on inferior, lateral, and medial gazes**. I will assess the **optic nerve function** by checking the visual acuity, relative afferent pupillary defect, color vision, and confrontational visual fields, and perform a **dilated fundal examination** for optic nerve atrophy or swelling for optic neuritis associated with multiple sclerosis. I will **examine the occiput** for neurosurgical scars for posterior cranial malformations, **check the oropharynx for synchronous movement of the palate** (oculopalatal myoclonus), examine for **cerebellar signs**, examine the patient's history for **drug use** and **alcoholism** and for **malignancy**, and refer the patient to the **internist for investigation** (paraneoplastic). Causes would include cervicomedullary junction **Arnold–Chiari malformation, cerebellar disease, drug such as lithium** and **phenytoin, multiple sclerosis, encephalitis, meningitis, diabetes mellitus,** and

paraneoplastic syndrome. Differentials include **oculopalatal myoclonus** secondary to brainstem stroke.

Note: **Oculopalatal myoclonus** is most commonly secondary to a **brain stem stroke**. Other causes include brain stem tumor, trauma, and multiple sclerosis. It is associated with a clicking sound which does not disappear on rest or sleep, and is associated with hypertrophy of the inferior olivary nucleus at the triangle of Guillain–Mollaret.

> **Q** **Question 22 OSCE Stem: Examination of One-and-a-Half Syndrome.**

On examination of this patient, there is **right gaze deficit with adduction deficit in the right eye and a left beating nystagmus in the left eye on left gaze** indicative of one-and-a-half syndrome with the lesion in the **right paramedian pontine recticular formation** and **medial longitudinal fasciculus**. I will check for **contiguous cranial nerves in the pontine region**; assess the **optic neuropathy** by checking for visual acuity, relative afferent pupillary defect, color vision, and confrontational visual field; and perform a **dilated fundal examination** for optic disc pallor and atrophy (indicative of **previous multiple sclerosis-associated optic neuritis**). Other causes include **trauma**, **stroke**, and **tumors**. I will confirm my diagnosis with **neuroimaging**. Differentials would include **myasthenia gravis**.

6. Miscellaneous

> **Q** **Question 23.1 Viva Stem: Elderly Patient presents with Chronic Red Eyes and some Discomfort (see Figure 5.21 showing Photo of Anterior Segment).**

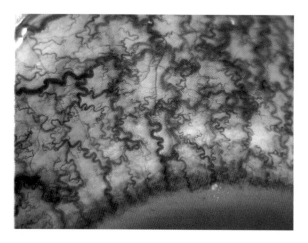

Figure 5.21 These are the classical cockscrew vessels seen in patients with carotid-cavernous fistula. Do note that patients can present acutely with a unilateral injected eye with unilateral proptosis.

This is the limited anterior segment photograph of the patient's right eye showing an **injected conjunctiva** with numerous **dilated cockscrew vessels** suggestive of carotid-cavernous fistula. I will examine the patient's history for the onset, duration, tinnitus, trauma, pain on eye movement, and ischemic risk factors. I will assess the **optic nerve function** by checking the visual acuity, relative afferent pupillary defect, confrontational visual fields, and color vision; check the **extraocular movements**; check for proptosis using a **Hertel's exophthalmometer; palpate for thrill** and **auscultate for bruit**; check for **lagophthalmos and Bell's reflex**; and check the anterior segment under the slit lamp for **exposure keratopathy** and for **flare in the anterior chamber more than cellular activity that might suggest anterior segment ischemia**. I will look at the iris for **rubeosis**; check for raised **intraocular pressure** and **pulsatile mires**; perform a **gonioscopy for angle closure, neovascularization,** and **blood in Schlemm's canal**; and perform a dilated fundal examination for **venous stasis retinopathy** or **central retinal vein occlusion, optic disc swelling**, or **increased cup-disc ratio**. I will check the contralateral eye, check the blood pressure, and check systemically for connective tissue disorders like Ehlers–Danlos syndrome. The gold standard investigation is a **four-vessel angiogram with digital subtraction**. Other modalities include **computer tomography of the orbit and brain with contrast and angiogram as well as magnetic resonance imaging of the orbit and brain with contrast and angiogram, and orbit Doppler ultrasound**. Management can be divided into systemic and ocular. I will co-manage the patient with the internist to monitor the associated vascular risk factors. If there are life-threatening complications such as **cortical venous drainage, I will refer the patient to the radiologist for definitive angiographic embolization**. Ocular management depends on the type as well as severity (see indications to treat). For **indirect fistulas, I will treat conservatively** and **monitor for spontaneous improvement**. This patient is likely to have a direct fistula. The definitive treatment would be angiographic embolization. I will treat associated complications like exposure keratopathy with lubricants, and glaucoma with glaucoma eye drops in the absence of contraindications. (Other treatment modalities include compression of carotids by contralateral hand and surgical ligation.)

Q Question 23.2 Describe the Image shown in Figure 5.22.

This photo is the T2-weighted axial cut of the magnetic resonance imaging scan through the brain and orbit showing the presence of **increased flow voids** (white arrow) with **convex bowing of the right cavernous sinus**. The **superior ophthalmic vein** is not well seen on this cut but it will likely be **dilated** in other cuts. There is **minimal proptosis** of the right globe and the rectus muscles are not significantly enlarged. There is no effacement of the gyri and no significant edema. The patient **has right carotid cavernous fistula with posterior cerebral drainage**.

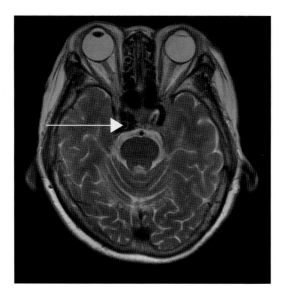

Figure 5.22 This is the T2-weighted magnetic resonance scan illustrating the presence of a right carotid cavernous fistula.

Q Question 23.3 What are the Sight-Threatening Complications?

The sight-threatening complications include **glaucoma, central retinal vein occlusion, exposure keratopathy,** and **compressive optic neuropathy**.

Q Question 23.4 What are the Life-Threatening Complications?

The life-threatening complications include **cerebral edema** and **venous infarction** secondary to **cortical venous drainage**.

Q Question 23.5 What are the Indications to Treat?

The indications to treat include **sight-threatening complications, severe bruit** and **life-threatening complications,** and **diplopia**.

Chapter 6

OCULOPLASTICS

Q Question 1.1 Viva Stem: How would you Manage a 5-year-old Child who constantly rubs the eyes and who has the following Features (see Figure 6.1)?

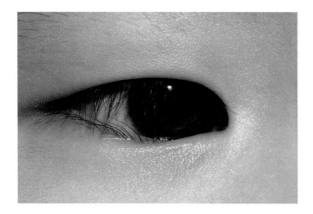

Figure 6.1 Right lower lid epiblepharon.

This is the anterior segment photograph of the right eye showing the presence of **right lower lid epiblepharon with an epicanthal fold**. The cornea appears **clear** and the **conjunctiva is white**. I will examine under the slit lamp for **corneal-lash touch**, stain the cornea with fluorescein for **punctuate epithelial erosions** and **epithelial defects**, and **flip the eyelids to look for papillae**. I will perform a dilated fundal examination for **retinal tears and detachment**, check the visual acuity, check the **cycloplegic refraction** for increased astigmatism, check the relative afferent papillary defect, and examine the fellow eye. I will get the patient's history from the parents with regard to the duration of symptoms and progression. Management will depend on the age of the patient and **severity of symptoms** and **signs**. For this patient, as the symptoms and signs appear **mild**, I will counsel the parents and recommend conservative treatment with **copious lubricants** and watch for **spontaneous improvements by the age of 7**. If symptoms and signs are severe (e.g. significant corneal scarring or epithelial defects), I will recommend surgical intervention with the **Hotz procedure for the lower lid epiblepharon**. In the meantime,

I will assess the child for **refractive ambylopia** (meridonial) and treat with full refractive correction.

Q **Question 1.2 What is the Hotz Procedure?**

The Hotz procedure involves excision of the excess overlying skin and orbicularis via a subciliary incision and placement of **tarsal fixation sutures** to evert the lashes.

Q **Question 2.1 Viva Stem: Parents bring in this 7-year-old Child (see Figure 6.2), worried about her Abnormal Head Posture during Reading. How will you manage this Patient?**

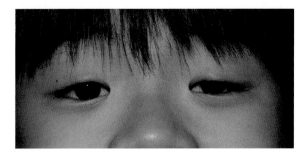

Figure 6.2 Bilateral congenital ptosis with the left lid obscuring the visual axis. This patient is at risk of developing amblyopia at the age of seven, hence necessitating early surgical intervention.

This is the partial facial photograph of the patient. The most obvious abnormality is the presence of **bilateral ptosis**, left worse than the right, in this young child. There is **obscuration of the visual axis** by the left lid. The eyes appear straight but I will lift up the eyelids to properly assess the **Hirschberg light reflex** in the left eye. The child is likely to have a **chin-up posture**. Notably, there is **absence of lid crease** bilaterally and no obvious masses are seen. I will check the visual acuity (looking for amblyopia), examine the pupils for anisocoria in light and dark (third cranial nerve palsy and Horner's syndrome) and relative afferent papillary defect, assess the extraocular movements, looking for limitations as well as lid retraction on downgaze (congenital ptosis). I will assess for **corneal sensation, lagophthalmos, Bell's reflex, and Marcus Gunn jaw winking phenomenon** (operative considerations). I will next measure the **palpebral aperture, marginal reflex distance 1,** and **levator function** (measure lid crease height if present) before completing my examination by checking the anterior segment, performing cycloplegic refraction of the child looking for **amblyopia** and **astigmatism**, and performing a dilated fundal examination.

This patient does not have features of blepharophimosis (such as shortened horizontal lid length, epicanthus inversus, telecanthus, hypertelorism, lateral ectropion, and flattened nasal bridge).

I will examine the patient's history for duration of ptosis and age of onset and whether it is progressive. I will ask if the child has difficulty seeing and whether the child is coping well in school. I will ask for a history of trauma especially during delivery, a family history of ptosis, **presence of diplopia**, and whether the ptosis is variable.

Note: In a child with bilateral ptosis, check for blepharophimosis. In scenarios with unilateral ptosis, check for Herring's effect by lifting the ptotic lid.

Q **Question 2.2 How would you Manage a PS stands for this Young Patient with the following: the Levator Palpebrae Superioris function is 3 mm Bilaterally; there is No Jaw Winking but she has Lid Retraction on Downgaze. Best Corrected Visual Acuity is OD 6/6 Plano/–0.50 × 180 and OS 6/12 –1.00/–2.00 × 170.**

This patient has **bilateral congenital ptosis** with left **meridonial** and **occlusion amblyopia**. Management of congenital ptosis depends on **presence of amblyopia** as well as **levator function**. This patient will require surgical intervention. In view of the **poor levator function** less than 4 mm, I will counsel the parents and recommend bilateral frontalis suspension using either autologous or donar **tensor fascia lata** in this age group or silicone rod/gortex, explaining to the parents that there would be **increased lid retraction on downgaze, lagophthalmos**, and **risk of exposure keratopathy**. To alleviate these, I will prescribe copious lubricants for the daytime and ointment at night and advise that she read with the neck flexed to reduce lid retraction. In the meantime, I will treat the amblyopia with **full refractive correction**, failing which I will consider **patching** the right eye for two hours a day.

Note: Sufficient length of tensor fascia lata is difficult to harvest in a child below three to four years old.

Q **Question 2.3 What are the Pre-Operative Considerations for Ptosis Surgery in a Child?**

There are several important considerations for a child. Preoperatively, visual acuity and cycloplegic refraction should be checked, underlying cause for the ptosis should be examined, and an assessment made of the child's fitness for operation and (use of anti-coagulants is more pertinent for adults). The following should also be checked: presence of **dry eyes, decreased corneal sensation, lagophthalmos, Bell's reflex**, and **presence of Herring's effect**.

Note: Landmark for harvesting of tensor fascia lata: 15 cm i.e. one hand breadth above the lateral femoral epicondyle, along a line connecting the anterior superior iliac crest to the lateral femoral condyle. At least 10 cm in length is required.

Q. Question 2.4 What is Marcus Gunn Jaw Winking and how would you Manage It?

Marcus Gunn jaw winking is a **synkinetic innervation of the pterygoid muscles and the levator by the trigeminal nerve.** If the wink excursion is **mild (less than 2 mm), mullerectomy** or **levator resection can be considered (treat ptosis). If it is 2 mm or more, then extirpation of the levator (including the medial and lateral horns of medial and lateral canthal ligament, upper 1/3 of tarsal, lid crease) with a frontalis sling is the treatment of choice.**

Q. Question 3 OSCE Stem: Examination of a Patient with Congenital Ptosis.

On examination of this patient, there is **partial ptosis in the right eye obscuring the visual axis.** There is **no abnormal head posture.** On lifting the lid, the eyes are straight in primary gaze with Hirschberg light reflex. There is **absence of the lid crease without a deep sulcus sign.** Examination shows that the **extraocular motility is full** but there is **lid retraction on downgaze.** Pupil examination is normal. This patient likely has right-sided congenital ptosis. I will check for **lagophthalmos, Bell's reflex, corneal sensation, and Marcus Gunn jaw winking.** I will also check for **Herring's sign as well as old photos, visual acuity and refraction (for amblyopia)** and perform measurements to check the **palpebral aperture, marginal reflex distance 1,** and **levator function.**

Q Question 4.1 Viva Stem: How would you Manage a 70-year-old Woman who presents with Gradual Obscuration of the Right Eye (see Figure 6.3)?

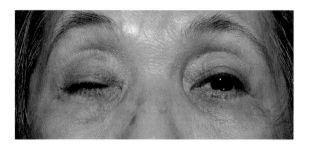

Figure 6.3 This patient presented with progressive ptosis on the right eye. She is otherwise well systemically. She has classical features of aponeurotic ptosis such as deep superior sulcus and increased lid crease.

This is the partial facial photo of the patient showing the presence of **right ptosis** that obscures the visual axis. There is **bilateral deep superior sulcus** with **increased lid crease height** on the right upper lid. I will lift up the right eye lid to **check for ocular deviation** using the Hirschberg light reflex. I will check the visual acuity; assess the pupils for **anisocoria** in light and dark as well as relative afferent papillary defect; assess the **extraocular movement** for limitation and increased ptosis on downgaze; **measure the palpebral aperture, marginal reflex distance 1, lid crease height,** and **levator function; check the corneal sensation, Bell's reflex,** and **Herring's sign,** and assess for signs of **ocular myasthenia** such as fatigability and poor obicularis strength.

I will examine the patient's history for duration of symptoms and whether they are acute or progressive. I will ask for presence of **diplopia, fatigability, variability, any history of trauma, orbital or ocular surgeries (e.g. cataract surgery), as well as contact lens wear (more appropriate for younger patients).**

Q **Question 4.2** How would you Manage a Patient who has Levator Palpebrae Superioris Function of 12 mm, Marginal Reflex Distance 1 of 2 mm and Increased Lid Crease?

This patient has severe right **aponeurotic ptosis**. I will **counsel and recommend ptosis repair with levator resection** (unilateral or **bilateral**) and inform the patient of the **risk of lagophthalmos, exposure keratopathy,** and **lid retraction on downgaze as well as contralateral ptosis secondary to Herring's law.**

Q **Question 4.3** How would you Perform the Surgery for the Patient in Question 4.2?

In view of the normal levator function but severe ptosis, I will perform **bilateral levator repair** for this patient under informed consent in the operating theater under **local anesthesia** (bilateral to attain better symmetry). Preoperatively I will check if the patient is on **anti-platelets or anti-coagulants**. I will stop the medications after consultation with the internist and restart immediately after the surgery.

I will **mark the incision site** as well as the **lid crease**, infiltrate with local anesthesia containing **lignocaine 2% and epinephrine 1:80000**. I will then incise the skin with a **Bard Parker 15 blade**, and **undermine** and **excise the obicularis** to expose the underlying orbital septum. I will then dissect through the orbital septum, by using a Weskott scissors held perpendicularly to create a **buttonhole**, looking for **fat prolapse**. I will then extend the defect medially and laterally. I will retract the preaponeurotic fat pad to expose the levator aponeurosis and identify the dehiscence from the tarsal plate. I will **disinsert the Muller's muscle** from the tarsal plate before attaching the levator back onto the **superior one-third of the tarsus using double armed 6/0 vicryl sutures**. I will aim to place **three sutures — medial, central**, and **lateral** (central suture is just medial to pupil), attaching the tarsus to the white band of the levator. I will repeat the same steps for the contralateral eye. Prior to closure, I will **adjust the height** and **contour** to maximize the symmetry between both eyes prior to excising the excess levator. I will close the skin wounds with 7/0 silk, incorporating the levator and fat pad to recreate the lid crease.

Q | **Question 5.1 Viva Stem: What is your Impression of a Middle-aged Patient who presents with Mild Ptosis, whose Levator Function is Normal, and who has a Miosed Pupil?**

This patient is likely to have **Horner's syndrome**. I will examine the patient's history for previous trauma to the neck, neck or thoracic surgery, and blocked ears or epistaxis. I will examine for other features of Horner's syndrome such as anhidrosis (triad of Horner's syndrome is anhidrosis, ptosis, and miosis, though anhidrosis occurs only if lesion is preganglionic), **inverse lid ptosis, relative enophthalmos**, hypotony, and heterochromia. I will check the cranial nerves, especially the extraocular movements and corneal sensation, perform a dilated fundal examination for disc swelling or pallor, examine for underlying cause — looking for long tract signs, nail clubbing and thenar wasting, tumors at the lung apex and carotid masses or thrill as well as cervical scars. I will perform pharmacological tests to **confirm the diagnosis and localize the lesion**. I will administer **cocaine 10% or apraclonidine 0.5% to confirm Horner's syndrome followed by hydroxyamphetemine 1% or phenylephrine 1% to determine the level of the lesion**. I will refer the patient to the otolaryngologist to exclude nasopharyngeal carcinoma, treat the underlying cause, and discuss with the patient regarding conservative or surgical management of the ptosis. An anterior or posterior approach can be considered for the ptosis repair. (If the patient has Horner's syndrome with ipsilateral neck scar, the patient might have previous tumor excision or carotid dissection repair.)

Foville Syndrome	Lateral Medullary Syndrome
• Fifth nerve — facial anesthesia	• Fifth nerve — loss of pain and temperature sensation in ipsilateral face and contralateral body
• Sixth nerve palsy combined with gaze palsy (PPRF)	• Eighth nerve — deafness
• Seventh nerve (nuclear or fascicular damage) — facial weakness	• Ninth and tenth nerve — dysarthria, dysphagia
• Eighth nerve — deafness	• Horner's syndrome
• Horner syndrome	• Cerebellar — nystagmus, ataxia

Dangerous Horner's Syndrome

1. Carotid dissection — painful Horner's syndrome
2. Lung cancer — pancoast tumor
3. Neuroblastoma in children
4. Cavernous sinus syndrome — associated with multiple cranial nerve palsies

Q Question 5.2 What Scans would you Order for the Patient in Question 5.1?

I would perform magnetic resonance of the **brain, orbit**, and **neck with angiogram with contrast as well as a computer tomography scan of the thorax with angiogram and contrast**.

Q Question 6.1 Viva Stem: How would you Manage a 70-year-old Patient who presents with Complaints of Recurrent Left Eye Redness and Discomfort (see Figure 6.4)?

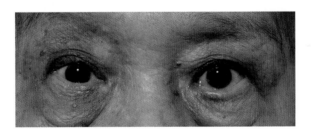

Figure 6.4 Causes of ectropion can be divided into involutional, paralytic, and cicatricial. This patient has left lower lid involutional ectropion with poor lid globe apposition, resulting in persistent ocular irritation.

This is the partial facial photo of the patient. The patient has left lower lid ectropion with poor lid globe apposition compared to the right eye. Otherwise the eyes appear straight on primary gaze, the conjunctiva is white, and the cornea is clear. The patient does not have obvious cicatricial lid changes in this photo nor brow ptosis that might suggest facial nerve palsy as a cause. I will check the visual acuity, stain the cornea looking for epitheliopathy, examine the conjunctiva and lid closely for cicatricial changes, check for features of facial nerve palsy (**loss of frontal creases, upper lid retraction, lagophthalmos, Bell's reflex, loss of nasolabial folds, and drooping of the angle of the mouth),** and assess for lagophthalmos and Bell's reflex. I will examine the lids, assessing for the integrity of medial and lateral canthal ligament and distraction, as well as conduct a snap back test.

I will examine the patient's history for eye redness and pain, duration of symptoms, and progression. I will also examine the patient's history for any previous trauma and for any previous acute facial asymmetry. Management for this patient can be divided into **conservative** and **surgical** treatment. Conservative treatment will include copious **lubricants** and ointments at night and topical broad-spectrum antibiotics in the absence of contraindications if the patient has significant corneal epitheliopathy. If the symptoms and signs are not relieved by medical treatment, I will offer surgical correction. **Surgical treatment** will depend on the **location and extent of the ectropion**. In this patient, the ectropion involves the **full width** of the lower lid. I will perform **full thickness pentagonal wedge resection** or **lateral tarsal strip procedure**.

Q **Question 6.2 How would you Perform the Surgery of your Choice?**

I will perform a **pentagonal wedge resection** for this patient under informed consent in the operating theater under local anesthesia (2% lignocaine with 1:80 000 adrenaline) and in sterile conditions. I will assess the **extent of horizontal lid shortening required** and mark my incision edges temporally with a skin marker. I will next place a **lid retraction suture** at the grey line using 4/0 silk (for counter traction), medial to my incision markings. I will **excise a full thickness pentagonal wedge using straight scissors**, with the sides **extending the entire height** of the inferior tarsal plate before connecting at the apex. I will suture the tarsal plates together using **6/0 vicryl interrupted sutures,** placing two to three sutures while ensuring **good alignment of the tarsus**. I will then appose the **grey line followed by the lash line** with **8/0 interrupted silk sutures, leaving the suture ends long** and avoiding a notch at the lid margin. I will then **close the skin with 8/0 interrupted silk sutures** while **incorporating the long suture ends**. (The method of closure is similar to the closure techniques used for lid lacerations that are full thickness or involving the lid margins.)

> **Key Points in OSCE Examination of a Patient with Facial Nerve Palsy**
>
> **Inspect**
>
> - forehead furrowing, brow ptosis, lower lid ectropion, asymmetrical blink reflex, presence of tarsorrhaphy
> - loss of nasal labial folds, dropping of corner of mouth
> - scar parotid — anterior/posterior auricular
>
> **Move/palpate**
>
> - loss of frontalis crease on upgaze, lift brows to look for lid retraction (secondary to unopposed CN III), poor orbicularis oculi strength with lagophthalmos, Bell's reflex
> - palpate for gold weight

- check cornea sensation
- smile/puff cheeks/teeth

Complete examination by doing the following

- perform optoscopy to look for vesicles → ramsay hunt
- check under slit lamp for punctal plug

Special tests

- Shirmer's
- take a history of hyperacusis
- assess taste of anterior 2/3 of tongue

- Look for aberrant facial nerve regeneration — crocodile tears, inverse Marcus gun.
- Examine under slit lamp to look for exposure keratopathy. Long tract signs: contralateral hemiparesis + cerebella signs → involvement of cerebellar pontine angle
- Check contiguous cranial nerves (5,6,7,8 — pons) → Cornea sensation V_1, eye movement especially cranial nerve VI, hearing cranial nerve VIII
- Refer otolaryngologist to rule out nasopharyngeal carcinoma

Causes of tearing in a patient with facial nerve palsy:

Punctal eversion, ectropion, reflex tearing due to dry eyes, aberrant regeneration

Note: localization of cranial nerves VII

- involvement of cranial nerves VI/cranial nerves V → brainstem
- Shirmer's (greater petrosal nerve) → above/on geniculate ganglion
- anterior 2/3 taste (chorda tympani) → below geniculate ganglion

---

Q **Question 7.1 Viva Stem: How would you Manage an 80-year-old Woman who presents with Recurrent Irritation in the Right Eye, and on Examination, was noted to have the Abnormalities shown in Figure 6.5?**

This is the anterior segment photo of the patient's right eye. The most obvious abnormality is the presence of **lower lid entropion** with **corneal lash touch** with associated **scaring** in the inferior nasal cornea. The patient **does not have cicatricial changes** on the skin. The conjunctiva is not injected, the cornea is otherwise clear, and the patient is pseudophakic. I will check the visual acuity, assess the **degree of horizontal laxity** by performing the **distraction and snap back test**, ask the patient to close her eyes to assess for

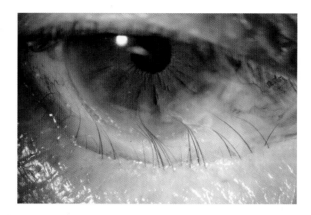

Figure 6.5 Involutional entropion is the most common form of entropion. Surgical correction should be considered when the patient has significant corneal epitheliopathy or discomfort which does not improve with topical lubricants.

overriding of the preseptal obicularis over the pretarsal obicularis, assess for **lower lid retractor dehiscence** by asking the patient to look down, palpate the tarsal plate to look for **tarsal plate atrophy**, and assess for **enophthalmos**. I would pull down the lid to look for **cicatricial conjunctival changes**, stain the cornea to look for epithelial defects, assess the cataract surgery wound (increased risk of endophthalmitis if the cataract surgery is recent) and examine the fellow eye.

I will examine the patient's history for eye redness, eye pain, duration of symptoms and progression, trauma, chemical injury, or previous ocular or lid surgeries.

> **Q** **Question 7.2 How do you Manage a Patient who does not have Cicatricial Changes but Distraction Test shows 8 mm and the Lid Fails to Snap Back after Anterior Distraction?**

This patient has involutional entropion with corneal scarring.

Management would depend on the **severity of the symptoms** and **signs** and whether patient is **medically well**. This patient will likely need **surgical intervention** in view of the corneal scarring. I will start with conservative treatment with **copious preservative-free lubricants with antibiotic cover**. If the patient is fit for surgery, options include **lateral tarsal strip procedure** or **full thickness pentagonal wedge resection** with **lower lid retractor repair**. If the patient is medically unfit for surgery, I will consider **temporizing lid everting sutures** with 6/0 double-armed vicryl sutures.

Q Questin 8.1 Viva Stem: How would you Perform a Dacryocystorhinostomy?

I will perform dacryocystorhinostomy under informed consent in the operating theater under regional and local anesthesia in sterile conditions. I will first **pack and spray nasal vasoconstrictors,** make a **1-cm incision 1 cm medial to the medical canthal angle,** dissect through the obicularis to reach the **anterior lacrimal crest, reflect the periosteum using Rollet periosteal elevator** to expose the lacrimal sac, reflect the lacrimal sac and create an **infracture using the Traquair periosteal elevator, complete the rhinostomy using Kerrison punch,** and infiltrate local anesthesia (lignocaine + adrenaline for hemostasis) into the lacrimal sac and nasal mucosa. I will then create an **H flap on both surfaces, closing the posterior flap with 6/0 vicryl,** following which I will insert a **00 Bowman probe into the cannaliculus** before cannulating using a bicannalicular **Bodkin's tube.** I will then close the **anterior flap (6/0 vicryl) and skin wound in layers (7/0 silk).** I will start the patient on **topical steroids** and **antibiotic eye drops, apply ointment to the skin wound, and advise the patient to refrain from exertion or blowing the nose.** I will **remove the suture after five days, remove the tube after three to six months, and repeat syringing.**

Methods to Reduce Hemorrhage

Preoperative

- Packing nose (cocaine) + spray with oxymethzoline

Intraoperative

- Bone wax for bone bleed
- Adrenaline-soaked gauze
- Lignocaine with adrenaline
- Reverse Trendelenburg position

Postoperative

- Pack the nasal space with Merocel
- Avoid hot food and drinks
- Avoid blowing of nose
- Maintain upright posture
- Common sites of bleed: nasal mucosa, bone, anterior ethmoidal artery, obicularis oculi

---

Note: In the event of significant post-operative bleeding, methods to reduce bleeding include the following: upright posture, chewing on ice cubes, nasal packing with adrenalin-soaked gauze. Refer the patient to the ENT specialist to perform cautery using the nasoendoscope, and to re-open and explore the wound in the operating theater.

Dacryocystorhinostomy is a surgical tear drainage procedure to create an anastomosis between the **lacrimal sac and the medial meatus** to bypass a nasolacrimal duct obstruction. It is indicated in patients with persistent epiphora with **complete nasolacrimal duct obstruction, congenital nasolacrimal duct obstruction, dacryocystocele**, and **recurrent nasolacrimal duct obstructions/dacryocystitis**.

The complications can be divided into intraoperative, and early and late postoperative stages. Intraoperative complications include trauma to the cannaliculus and medial rectus, globe trauma, hemorrhage and cerebrospinal fluid leakage/base of skull fracture. Early postoperative complications include hemorrhage, cerebrospinal fluid leakage, and infection. Late complications include stent infection, stent migration or extrusion, **sump syndrome** (osteotomy is too small and high), restenosis or persistance of epiphoria.

Q **Question 8.3 When are Stents Indicated?**

Stents are indicated in **repeat dacryocystorhinostomy (recurrent)**, when there is **excessive bleeding intraoperatively** or when there is **excessive scarring** noted, and in patients with **cannalicular obstruction**.

Q **Question 8.4 What are the Indications for Endoscopic Dacryocystorhinostomy?**

I will perform endoscopic dacryocystorhinostomy in **young patients who want to avoid visible scars**, in patients with concomitant **treatable nasal pathologies such as polyps**, and in patients with **active dacryocystitis**.

Q **Question 9.1 Viva Stem: How would you Manage a 30-year-old Woman who was punched in the Face and presents with Complaints of Double Vision (see Figure 6.6)?**

This is the partial facial photograph of the patient showing left periorbital hematoma involving the upper and lower lid with associated periorbital swelling. The eyes are straight on Hirschberg light reflex and the left eye is not proptotic. The patient does not have any obvious lid nor cannalicular injuries.

Principles would be to first exclude **life-threatening injuries** and subsequently **sight-threatening injuries**. I will examine the patient's history for the timing of injury, loss of

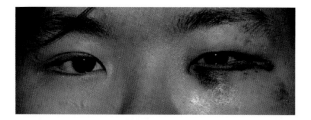

Figure 6.6 This patient suffered blunt trauma with resultant floor fracture. Patients with oculocardiac reflex will require urgent surgical intervention.

consciousness, blurring of vision, and presence of diplopia. After excluding life-threatening injuries, I will assess for **optic nerve function by checking visual acuity, relative afferent pupillary defect, color vision, and confrontational visual fields**. I will check for **orbital rim step deformities, crepitus, temporal mandibular joint malocclusion**, and **proptosis**, as well as check for **infraorbital anesthesia**. I will then examine **extraocular movements** for restriction and oculocardiac reflex. I will check the **anterior segment** for evidence of lacerations or abrasions, globe perforation, intraocular pressure, whether the anterior chamber is formed or abnormally deep, presence of cellular activity or hyphema, sphincter rupture, iridodialysis, cataract, and subluxation of the lens. I will perform a **dilated fundal examination** for vitreous hemorrhage, commotion retinae, retinal tears, detachment or dialysis, and disc swelling. I will perform a facial bone X-ray looking for **fractures, tear drop sign and opacification of the maxillary sinus**, and do a **computer tomography of the orbits with 1-mm fine cuts**.

> **Q** **Question 9.2 A Computer Tomography Scan was performed as shown in Figure 6.7. The Patient has Restricted Extraocular Motility without Oculocardiac Reflex. How would you Manage such a Patient and what are the Indications for Surgical Repair?**

This is the **bone-window computer tomography scan** of the orbits illustrating the presence of isolated left inferior floor fracture with **herniation of orbital contents inferiorly**. The inferior rectus is **displaced inferiorly but it is not entrapped**. This patient has left inferior floor fracture without entrapment.

The indications for orbital floor repair include (1) urgent indications such as **white eye blow out fracture (ischemia)** and **ocular cardiac reflex**, (2) non-urgent indications such as **diplopia on primary or downgaze, enophthalmos of at least 2 mm, fracture extending more than 50% of the anterior-posterior length of the orbit, or significant hypoglobus and entrapment**.

In this patient, I will perform orbital floor fracture repair about one to two weeks after the initial injury for swelling to subside. In the meantime, I will advise the patient to **refrain**

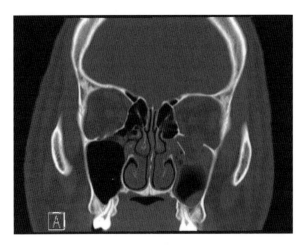

Figure 6.7

from blowing of nose and exertion, and start the patient on broad spectrum oral anti-biotics in the absence of contraindications. I will perform preoperative baseline Hess binocular single vision charting and facial photos in nine cardinal positions of gaze as well as a preoperative fitness workup.

Q Question 9.3 What are the Mechanisms of Floor Fracture?

Floor fracture develops as a result of **increased hydrostatic pressure** due to compression of the globe axially, **direct trauma to the orbital rim with transmission of force resulting in buckling of the orbital floor,** and **globe wall displacement**.

Q Question 9.4 How would you Repair the Floor Fracture?

I will perform floor fracture repair under informed consent under general anesthesia in sterile conditions. I will perform **lateral canthotomy** and **inferior cantholysis,** and **enter the orbital cavity via a transconjunctival approach,** dissecting through the **preseptal plane to reach the orbital rim** and **reflect the periosteum**. I will use a **malleable retractor to retrieve all the orbital contents** and **to assess the extent of the floor fracture**. I will then **size and insert an integrable implant** (e.g. porous polyethylene PPE or osteomesh), ensuring that it is well supported, and check for residual entrapment using forced duction test and subsequently **close the wound in layers**. I will admit the patient postoperatively for **close monitoring of relative afferent pupillary defect and visual acuity**.

> **Q** **Question 10.1** Viva Stem: A Patient has suffered Blunt Trauma to the Face and presents with Pain and Blurring of Vision. On Examination, it was found that he has Unilateral Proptosis with Chemosis and an Intraocular Pressure of 60. What is your Impression and how would you Manage such a Patient?

This patient has **retrobulbar hemorrhage which is an ocular emergency**. The definitive treatment would be an urgent **lateral canthotomy** and **inferior cantholysis**. In the meantime, I will start the patient on **topical glaucoma eye drops and intravenous mannitol** in the absence of contraindications. I will perform the procedure under informed consent in the treatment room, **infiltrate with local anesthesia in sterile conditions**. I will first clamp the lateral canthal tendon with an artery forceps, then cut using a straight scissors till I reach the **lateral orbital rim**. I will isolate the **inferior crus of the lateral canthal tendon** by strumming the lower lid with a **curved artery forceps**. I will then **cut the inferior crus vertically with the straight scissors** till I reach the **orbital rim** and the lower lid is adequately mobilized. I will then recheck and monitor the intraocular pressure closely subsequently.

> **Q** **Question 10.2** How do you Tell that the Surgery in Question 10.1 was Successful?

There will be a **gush of blood** with associated **globe retraction** backwards into the orbit.

> **Q** **Question 11.1** Viva Stem: Describe the Photograph in Figure 6.8 which shows a Patient who was accidentally hit by a glass panel. (The Right Eye has been Pharmacologically Dilated.) How will you Manage such a Patient?

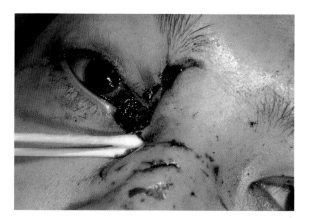

Figure 6.8 Canalicular lacerations are extremely challenging to manage and surgical treatment should not be delayed. This patient will require prolonged intubation with a stent to maintain the patency of the canaliculus.

This is the partial facial photo of the patient showing the presence of a **large vertical laceration involving the right upper and lower lid along the medial canthus that appears medial to the punctum**. There are multiple superficial linear lacerations along the nasal bridge. The eye is injected with subconjunctival hemorrhage medially. The cornea is clear and the **globe grossly looks intact** without prolapse of uveal tissue and no foreign body, but I will examine carefully under the slit lamp to look for areas of perforation and **involvement of the canaliculus**. I will first exclude life-threatening injuries, assess the optic nerve function by checking the visual acuity, relative afferent pupillary defect, color vision, and confrontational visual field, pull down the lower lid, flip the upper lid, and sweep to look for foreign bodies. I will then perform a dilated fundal examination to exclude intraocular foreign body, retinal tear/detachment and disc swelling.

This patient has both **upper and lower lid laceration with likely canaliculus involvement**.

I will take a history with regard to the timing and onset of the injury, whether the glass panel shattered, use of protective eyewear, any loss of consciousness, whether there was removal of foreign bodies and blurring of vision, and the time of the patient's last meal and drink.

Q **Question 11.2 How would you Identify the Distal Portion of a Lacerated Canaliculus?**

There are several methods to help identify the distal end of the canaliculus. Firstly, I will examine under **direct visualization with illumination**, following which I can examine under the microscope. If that fails, I can **instill topical phenylephrine eye drops** looking for the **calamari sign**. Other options include (1) **flooding the area with normal saline**, compressing the lacrimal sac, and identifying the area of **bubbling** (indicates site of distal end), and (2) **injecting fluorescein dye** from the superior canaliculus and looking for leakage from the distal end of the lower canaliculus (assuming that the distal end of the upper canaliculus can be isolated in this case).

Note: Pigtail probe is viable only if the patient has a common canaliculus. It will not be a suitable option for the patient unless the distal section of the upper canaliculus is found.

> Repair of canalicular lacerations:
> - Identify distal lacerated end.
> - Intubate with mono-canalicular stent e.g. mini-Monoka or bi-canalicular stent e.g. Crawford tube.
> - Re-attach the lacerated ends by apposing the pericanalicular tissues with 8/0 vicryl.

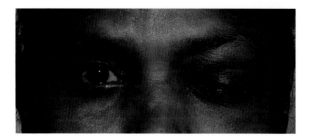

Figure 6.9 This patient has left orbital cellulitis with a complete mechanical ptosis secondary to lid swelling. A third cranial nerve palsy secondary to orbital apex abscess or cavernous sinus thrombosis should still be excluded in such patients. In addition, mucomycosis as a cause for orbital cellulitis should be excluded in diabetic patients.

This is the facial photo of the patient showing left **upper and lower lid erythema** and **swelling with complete ptosis**. No external wounds or punctum are seen. I will lift up the eye lids to look for proptosis, ocular deviation, and injection as well as chemosis. The right eye appears normal and non-proptosed (proptosis of contralateral eye would indicate cavernous sinus thrombosis, especially in the presence of a complete ptosis). This patient is likely to have orbital cellulitis which is both a sight-and potentially life-threatening condition. Differentials include **preseptal cellulitis, orbital inflammatory disease,** or **a ruptured dermoid cyst**.

I will examine the patient's history for **duration of the symptoms, progression, whether there is associated diplopia, any recent trauma, localized swelling, dental procedures,** and **other causes of immunosuppression** or **history of sinusitis**. I will check the **vital signs** and assess the **optic nerve function** by checking the visual acuity, relative afferent pupillary defect, color vision, and confrontational fields. I will investigate the **source of infection** such as cuts as well as **palpate for styes**. I will check the **extraocular movement**, examine the contiguous cranial nerves such as **corneal sensation**, examine the anterior segment for **exposure keratopathy**, check the **intraocular pressure**, and perform a dilated fundal examination for **disc swelling** and **choroidal folds**. I will check the **full blood count, erythrocyte sedimentation rate, C-reactive protein, blood cultures, chest X-ray,** and **urine cultures**. I will admit the patient, monitor the **visual acuity** and **relative afferent pupillary defect** as well as **vitals closely**. I will start the patient on intravenous **cloxacillin 500 mg every six hours, amoxicillin clavalunic acid 1.2 g every eight hours, metronidazole 500 mg every eight hours if there is significant sinusitis,** and **topical**

broad-spectrum antibiotic drops in the absence of contraindications. I will perform a **computer tomography scan with contrast with fine cuts of the orbit** and **paranasal sinus** and co-manage the patient with the otolaryngologist and infectious disease specialist. If there is a **large orbital or subperiosteal abscess, or if the abscess is not responding to treatment or there is significant compressive optic neuropathy, I will then consider surgical drainage**.

> Indications for drainage of orbital abscess:
>
> Nine years or older, large abscess, lack of response to medical treatment (e.g. increasing proptosis, worsening relative afferent pupillary defect, worsening vision), significant optic nerve compression, large non-medial subperiosteal abscess, suspicion of anaerobic infection
>
> Note: Children younger than nine years old — mono-organism. Patients that are at least nine years old — multi-organisms. Adults are usually staph/strep while children frequently grow hemophilus.

Q Question 13.1 Viva Stem: Describe the Photo shown in Figure 6.10.

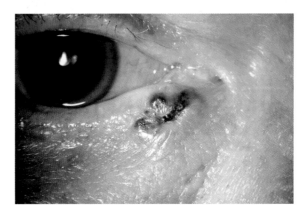

Figure 6.10 Basal cell carcinoma is locally invasive and most commonly arises from the lower lid. Medial lesions are more worrisome due to their potential of intracranial spread.

This is the color photograph of the patient's right eye, showing a lesion in the medial lower lid that is **pigmented**, pearly in appearance resembling a **rodent ulcer** with rolled edges with associated **madarosis** but sparing the lid margin without focal ectropion. It is small and occupying less than one-third of the width of the lower lid. There is **absence of active**

bleeding. It is adjacent to the punctum. I will confirm involvement by performing a **syringing procedure**. I will check the contralateral eye; assess the **optic nerve function** by checking the visual acuity, relative afferent pupillary defect, color vision, and confrontational visual field; check the optic nerve for disc swelling or atrophy; check the **extraocular movements** and presence of **proptosis** by using Hertel's exophthalmolmeter; examine for **regional lymphadenopathy (rare in basal cell carcinoma)**, examine the patient's history for duration and progression, radiation, excessive sunlight exposure, any skin cancers, and examine the family history for cancer. This patient has basal cell carcinoma of the medial lower lid of the left eye.

Q Question 13.2 Describe the Photo shown in Figure 6.11.

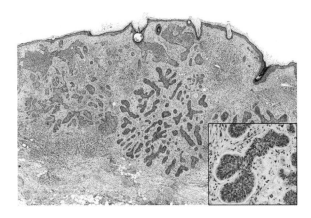

Figure 6.11 Histological slide of basal cell carcinoma (H + E, x20 magnification).

This histological slide shows the low-power microscopy revealing irregular islands of **basaloid cells** continuous with the basal layer of the epidermis, **invading into the underlying dermis**. The epidermis is intact without evidence of ulceration in this slide. Inset photo shows an irregular **nest** of uniform **hyperchromic basophilic** basaloid cells with **peripheral nuclear palisading** and a **cleft between the nest and surrounding stroma**.

Q Question 13.3 How would you Treat the Patient in Figure 6.10?

Principles of management is to obtain confirmatory histology by incisional biopsy, followed by excisional biopsy and repair of lid margin.

I will first confirm the diagnosis by performing an **incisional biopsy**. Once confirmed, the treatment can be divided into **systemic** and **ocular**. Systemically, I will co-manage the patient with a dermatologist and perform a **computer tomography scan of the orbits with contrast to look for extension**. Ocular management will depend on extent of the lesion. In this patient, I will first perform an incisional biopsy to confirm the diagnosis followed by wide excision with **3-mm** clear margins **fixed in paraffin** followed by reconstruction of the lower lid. As lesion size with clear margin excision is less than one-third the horizontal lid length, I will perform a lateral canthotomy and direct closure of the defect. (Other scenarios include the following: (1) As lesion size is between one-third and half of the horizontal lid length, I will reconstruct using the Tenzel semicircular flap technique. (2) As lesion size is greater than half the horizontal lid length, I will reconstruct using lid-sharing technique such as the **Hughes posterior lamellar tarsoconjunctival flap technique**.)

Note: 3-mm clear margins is required for basal cell carcinoma. 5-mm clear margins are required for squamous cell carcinoma, sebaceous cell carcinoma, and melanoma.

Incisional biopsy: infiltrate with small amounts of local anesthetic; incise and remove adequate tissue at edge of lesion with adjacent normal skin; avoid crushing the specimen when holding with the forceps.

Q **Question 13.4 What is the Problem of using a 3-mm Clear Margin Excision?**

There might be **significant loss of tissue, primary repair might be difficult**, and patient might require a flap. In addition, there might be **extension beyond the 3-mm clear margin**, especially for the sclerosing/morpheaform carcinoma.

Q **Question 13.5 What Alternative Surgical Treatment is available for this Patient?**

Moh's micrographic excision can be performed or cryotherapy for small lesions.

Q **Question 13.6 Which Syndrome is Basal Cell Carcinoma associated with Systemically?**

Systemically, basal cell carcinoma is associated with **Gorlin-Goltz syndrome**.

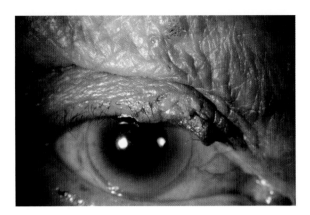

Figure 6.12 Sebaceous cell carcinoma can present as recurrent chalazion. A high index of suspicion is required to make an early diagnosis.

This is the photograph of the patient's right upper lid showing a **yellowish irregular mass involving and destroying the lid margin** with **central ulceration** and **madarosis** involving about a quarter of the lid width. I will examine the rest of the eye for **satellite nodules**; **flip the eyelid to assess for extension** and presence of papillary conjunctivitis; examine the fellow eye; assess **the optic nerve function** by checking the visual acuity, color vision, confrontational visual fields, and relative afferent pupillary defect; check the optic disc for disc swelling, **extraocular movements,** and **proptosis** using a Hertel's exophthalmometer; check for **regional lymphadenopathy**; examine the patient's history for duration and progression as well as radiation, excessive sun exposure, smoking, and any skin cancers; and examine the family history for cancers and history of recurrent blepharitis or chalazions. This patient is likely to have sebaceous cell carcinoma. Differentials include squamous cell and basal cell carcinoma.

Q **Question 14.2 How would you Treat this Patient in Question 14.2?**

Principles of management indicate obtaining confirmatory histology by incisional biopsy, followed by excisional biopsy and repair of lid margin.

I will first confirm the diagnosis by performing an incisional biopsy. Once confirmed, the treatment can be divided into **systemic** and **ocular** management. Systemically, I will co-manage the patient with a dermatologist (an oncologist if it is metastatic) and perform a **computer tomography scan of the orbits with contrast to look for extension**. Ocular management will depend on extent of the lesion. If it is localized, I will first perform a **wide excision with 5-mm** clear margins, send **fresh for Oil Red O stain** and **conjunctival map biopsy** inferiorly and superiorly followed by reconstruction of the lower lid. As lesion size with 5-mm clear margins is likely within one-third to half the horizontal lid length, I will reconstruct using the **Tenzel semicircular flap technique**. (Separate scenario: As lesion size is greater than half the horizontal lid length, I will reconstruct using lid sharing techniques such as **Cutler Beard full thickness lower lid advancement** [For upper lid lesions].) If the conjunctival map biopsy is positive, I will proceed to a sentinel lymph node biopsy, following which the patient will need a systemic review if it is positive as well.

Anterior Lamella (Skin Graft)	Posterior Lamella (Mucosal Graft)
• Adjacent skin, opposite lid skin, other eye • Retroauricular skin • Supraclavicular skin • Inner arm skin	• Adjacent tarsal plate, opposite tarsal plate, other eye • Hard palate (less suitable for upper lid)/buccal mucosa • Ear cartilage • Perichondrium

Features of Malignancy

- Ulceration
- Irregular distinct borders
- Dilated telangiectatic blood vessels
- Ectropion from skin contracture
- Firm induration
- Thickened eyelid margin
- Loss of eyelashes
- Palpable preauricular nodes
- Proptosis
- Ptosis
- Restricted ocular motility

Note: Lid-sharing procedures are not suitable for only-eyed patients and children (due to occlusion amblyopia).

Q **Question 14.3 What is the Mechanism of Spread of Sebaceous Cell Carcinoma?**

Sebaceous cell carcinoma can spread via direct extension, hematogenous spread, lymphatics, or pagetoid spread

Q **Question 14.4 Describe the Photo in Figure 6.13.**

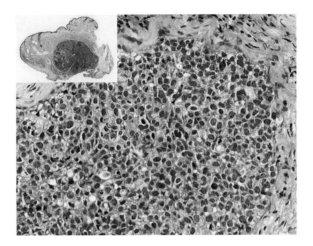

Figure 6.13   Histopathological slide of sebaceous gland carcinoma. Lipid is contained within the vacuoles. (H+ E, x 600 magnification)

This histopathology slide under high power microscopy shows sheets of malignant, pleomorphic hyperchromatic basophilic cells with some vacuolated cytoplasm (foamy appearance). Inset photo shows a lobulated tumor within the dermis of the eyelid.

Q **Question 14.5 Which Syndrome is Sebaceous Gland Carcinoma associated with Systemically?**

Systemically, sebaceous gland carcinoma is associated with **Muir-Torre syndrome**.

Q **Question 15.1 Viva Stem: Describe the Photo in Figure 6.14 which shows a Patient who presents with Blurring of Vision and Eye Discomfort.**

This photo of the patient shows an attentive gaze with **bilateral lid retraction** with **superior and inferior scleral show**. Hirschberg reflex is **deviated superiorly** in the right eye and there appears to be **proptosis** bilaterally. I will confirm by using a Hertel's exophthalmometer. There is **swelling** of the upper lids and **erythema** of the lower lids. Both eyes are injected without chemosis. The left **caruncle is injected and swollen**. Both corneas appear relatively clear in the presence of fluorescein staining. I will check the **extraocular**

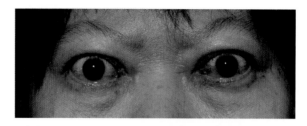

Figure 6.14 When approaching a patient with thyroid eye disease, it is important to determine the activity and severity of the condition. This will provide the framework which you can use to organize your answers. The patient has active thyroid eye disease with moderate severity and will require immunosuppression.

movements for limitation as well as **lid lag on downgaze**. I will ask the patient to close the eyes to look for **lagophthalmos** as well as **Bell's reflex** and check the **corneal sensation**. I will palpate to feel for **thrill**, assess resistance toward **retropulsion** and auscultate for **bruit**. I will assess the **optic nerve function** by checking the visual acuity, relative afferent pupillary defect, color vision, and confrontational visual field. I will examine the **anterior segment under the slit lamp**, looking for exposure keratopathy, superior limbic keratitis, conjunctival injection, and chemosis, as well as caruncular or plicae inflammation; check the intraocular pressures on straight gaze and upgaze as well as the lens status; and perform a **dilated fundal examination** for disc swelling or pallor, increased cup-disc ratio, and choroidal folds. I will examine systemically for goiter, palmar erythema, atrial fibrillation, and pretibial myxedema. I will examine the patient's history for hyperthyroidism, duration and progression, treatment, previous use of radioactive iodine, smoking, blurring of vision, diplopia, and pain at rest or on eye movements. The most likely diagnosis is bilateral active thyroid eye disease with at least moderate severity.

Q | **Question 15.2** What Clinical Grading will you use for Grading of the Activity of Thyroid Eye Disease?

I will use the **Clinical Activity Score** to grade the activity. On acute presentation, at least **three out of seven** points will be classified as active. These points are conjunctival injection, chemosis, lid erythema, lid swelling, caruncular or plicae inflammation, and ocular pain at rest or on movements.

If the patient has been on follow-up for at least three months, at least **four out of ten points** will be classified as active. The additional three points to the previously mentioned criteria include visual acuity **decreasing by at least one line, proptosis increasing by at least 2 mm, and increasing limitation of extraocular movements by at least eight degrees.**

EUGOGO Classification — Severity		
Mild	**Moderate**	**Severe**
• Lid retraction < 2 mm • Exophthalmos < 3 mm above normal • Mild soft tissue involvement • Transient or no diplopia • Corneal exposure responsive to lubricants	• Lid retraction > 2 mm • Exophthalmos > 3 mm • Constant diplopia • Moderate/severe soft tissue involvement • Symptomatic disease affecting functioning	One or more: • severe exposure keratopathy • compressive optic neuropathy

Q Question 15.3 Describe the Photo in Figure 6.15.

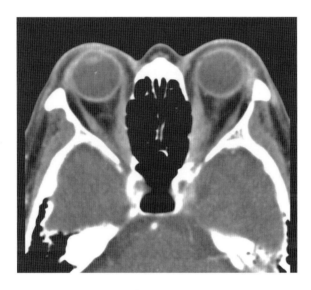

Figure 6.15

This is a computer tomography scan through the **orbits, axial cut** in the **soft tissue window**. There is presence of **bilateral proptosis** with **fusiform enlargement** of bilateral medial rectus with **tendon-sparing**. It is associated with **fat stranding** and possible **apical crowding**. The globe is not tented and the lacrimal gland is not well visualized. Grossly, there is absence of orbital wall remodeling in this patient.

This patient has severe active disease which is a **sight-threatening condition**. Management can be divided into **systemic** and **ocular**. Systemically, I will co-manage the patient with the endocrinologist to control the thyroid function. Ocular-wise, the **mainstay of treatment is immunosuppression**. In the absence of contraindications, I will admit the patient for **presteroid workup** and start the patient on intravenous methylprednisolone **1 g every other day/every day for three days (maximum lifetime dose of 8 g — another alternative regime is 500 mg every other day for three days)** while monitoring the patient closely. I will also start systemic oral immunosuppression with steroid-sparing agents. I will perform **surgical decompression** for the patient if the **steroid therapy fails** and **if systemic steroid therapy is contraindicated or has intolerable side effects**. I will also start the patient on copious amounts of preservative-free lubricants and broad-spectrum topical preservative-free antibiotics in the meantime.

Note: Intravenous methylprednisolone is indicated for both severe and active moderate thyroid eye disease.

Surgical decompression: (1) fat decompression (2) bony decompression

- Decompression for exposure keratopathy: remove lateral wall and fat.
- Decompression for compressive optic neuropathy: remove **posterior medial wall** and **medial floor** which are closest to the optic nerve.

Timing of surgical decompression:

- In compressive optic neuropathy, decompress if there is no improvement after two weeks post-intravenous methylprednisolone.
- In patients with disfiguring proptosis with exposure keratopathy, attempt two to three cycles of intravenous methylprednisolone one month apart. Decompress if there is no improvement.

Q **Question 15.5** What are the Indications for Surgical Decompression?

The indications include **compressive optic neuropathy, severe disfiguring proptosis, severe exposure keratopathy,** and **failure of or contraindication to medical decompression**.

Q **Question 15.6** When will you Consider Radiotherapy?

I will consider radiotherapy in patients with active moderate or severe thyroid eye disease with **restrictive myopathy,** especially if surgical or medical decompression is contraindicated.

(Radiotherapy is indicated in active moderate or severe thyroid disease with restrictive myopathy but not for acute compressive optic neuropathy. Contraindications include patients younger than 35 years old, history of skin cancer, and presence of ischemic risk factors.)

Q **Question 15.7** What are the Blinding Conditions in Thyroid Eye Disease?

Blinding conditions include **glaucoma, compressive optic neuropathy,** and **exposure keratopathy**.

Q **Question 15.8** How would you Manage a Patient who is Inactive now with Diplopia?

Management can be divided into systemic and ocular. Systemically I will co-manage the patient with an internist to control the thyroid function. Ocular management can be divided into conservative and surgical management. Conservative management will include prisms, botulinum injection, and Bangerter foils. Surgical management is indicated when there is **diplopia in primary or downgaze,** and **stable inactive thyroid eye disease with stable myopathy for at least six months**. I will perform **recession** of the rectus muscles to match ductions of both eyes with adjustable hang back technique (similar to Duane's syndrome — only recess and never resect).

Q **Question 15.9** What are the Risk Factors for Thyroid Eye Disease?

Patients who are at higher risk are **elderly patients, male patients, Caucasian patients, smokers, and those who suffer from vascular risk factors like hypertension, poor control of hyperthyroidism, hypothyroidism secondary to radioactive iodine treatment, rapid progression,** and **high antibody titers.**

Q Question 15.10 What is the Pathophysiology of Thyroid Eye Disease?

Thyroid eye disease can be divided into the acute and chronic phase. Acutely there is infiltration by **acute inflammatory cells with deposition of glycosaminoglycans (GAG)** with hypertrophy of the extraocular muscles and proliferation of soft tissues like orbital fat and lacrimal glands. Chronically there is **fibrosis** and **infiltration by chronic inflammatory cells**.

Q Question 15.11 What are Potential Complications of Orbital Decompression?

Complications can be divided into **intraoperative and postoperative**. Intraoperative complications include **globe trauma** and **perforation, trauma to rectus muscles, cerebrospinal fluid leak, trauma to optic nerve, ciliary ganglion,** and **infraorbital nerve and retrobulbar hemorrhage**. Postoperative complications include **cerebrospinal fluid leakage, retrobulbar hemorrhage, infections, silent sinus syndrome, diplopia, hypoglobus,** and **lid position changes**.

Q Question 16 OSCE Viva: Examination of the Patient shown in Figure 6.16.

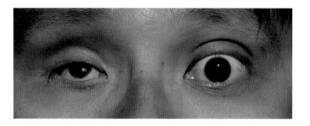

Figure 6.16 This patient underwent right enucleation for the treatment of retinoblastoma during his childhood. He has typical features of post-enucleation socket syndrome such as ptosis and enophthalmos.

On examination of this patient, he has a right prosthetic eye. There is associated **ptosis with deep superior sulcus** and **presence of lower lid ectropion**. The prosthesis is displaced posteriorly and rotated superiorly. I will confirm the enophthalmos with Hertel's exophthalmometer. There is associated **horizontal lid laxity with positive distraction** (> 6 mm away from globe) and **snap back test**. I will examine the **extraocular motility**. There is limitation of the motility of the right ocular prosthesis. I will examine under the slit lamp, pulling down the lower lid to assess for **forniceal shortening; flip the upper lid to look for papillary conjunctivitis; ask the patient to remove the prosthesis to assess the state**

of the prosthesis and underlying mucosa; look for infection or discharge; and assess for presence, extrusion, or exposure of the orbital implant. In summary, this patient has post-enucleation socket syndrome. Externally there are no lid or facial scars to suggest previous trauma. I will examine the **fellow eye to look for a cause** and **presence of sympathetic ophthalmia**. I will examine the patient's history for previous trauma, ocular malignancies, and infections.

> Important differentials to consider in a patient with enophthalmos:
>
> - Long-standing orbital varix
> - Post-enucleation socket syndrome
> - Previous orbital decompression surgery
> - Previous severe inflammation e.g. orbital inflammatory disease/infection/radiotherapy
> - Silent sinus syndrome
> - Previous orbital floor fracture
> - Malignancy e.g. scirrhous breast cancer, prostate cancer
> - Phthsis bulbi
> - Pseudoenophthalmos

Q **Question 16.2 How do you Manage Post-Enucleation Socket Syndrome?**

Management of post-enucleation socket syndrome is complicated and requires a stepwise approach. First, I will treat any associated **infection** with topical antibiotics in the absence of contraindications and irrigate the area. Next, I will treat orbital volume and implant issues. If there is insufficient orbital **volume**, I will implant **dermal fat graft** or **replace with a larger implant**. If there is exposure or extrusion of the implant, management depends on the size of the defect. If the defect is small, I will attempt direct closure. If it is large, a buccal mucosa patch graft will be required. If it is very large, a dermal fat graft might be required with smoothening of the orbital implant surface in cases of exposure. Next, I will correct **conjunctival deficiency with conjunctival or buccal mucosa transplant**. I will then treat lid abnormalities such as entropion and ectropion and ptosis, and finally treat any prosthetic issues.

Q **Question 16.3 How would you Perform an Evisceration?**

I will perform an evisceration under informed consent in the operating theater under **regional anesthesia** and in sterile conditions with **three consultant signatures (depends**

on institutional practice). I will incise the cornea at the limbus from **3 to 9 o'clock using a Beaver blade**, completing the remaining incision using **corneal scissors**, holding the cornea using **Jayles forceps**, and retracting the scleral with **Kilner hooks**. I will remove the intraocular contents **by entering through the suprachoroidal space using a cyclo-dialysis spatula**. I will **remove remnant tissues with a cellulose sponge and send the contents for cultures and/or histopathology**. I will then pack with **adrenalin-soaked ribbon gauze to achieve hemostasis** before treating **with 100% alcohol (to remove any residual choroid to prevent sympathetic ophthalmia, taking care not to affect the surrounding structures, followed by gentamicin wash**. I will **repack with ribbon gauze** and put on a **conformer followed by pressure bandage**, aiming for **a secondary orbital implantation as well as prosthesis implantation one to two months later**.

(If primary orbital implant is intended, create 360 degrees conjunctival peritomy, perform posterior sclerostomy, enter the posterior tenon's space, size and place implant — usually 20–22 mm diameter implant. Attach rectus muscles to the implant/wrap with 6/o vicryl. Posterior relaxing incisions might be needed followed by (1) closing of the sclera with double breasted method (2) closing tenon's using 6.0 vicryl and (3) conjunctival closure with 8/o vicryl in layers.)

Prosthesis implantation: six weeks to two months post-enucleation/evisceration Dermis fat graft: umbilicus/buttocks	
Inert (non-integrating) (non-porous)	**Bioreactive (integrating) (porous)**
• Requires scleral shell, temporalis fascia or fascia lata • Glass, silicon, plastics, acrylate *Advantages* • Decrease host response • Decrease exposure • Cheap *Disadvantages* • Increase extrusion • Cannot attach extraocular muscles • Poor motility	• Hydroxyapaptite, porous polypropylene, med pore *Advantages* • Decrease extrusion • Attach extraocular muscles • Good motility *Disadvantages* • Increase host response • Increase exposure • Expensive

Q **Question 17 OSCE Stem: Examine this Patient (see Figure 6.17).**

On examination of this patient, he appears to have a right-sided **proptosis** with superior and inferior scleral show. The right eye is deviated nasally on Hirschberg test suggestive of non-axial proptosis. The right conjunctiva appears injected. The lids are neither edematous nor erythematous. The lacrimal region is slightly swollen. There is absence of temporal fullness. I will confirm the proptosis by checking from the back. This confirms the presence

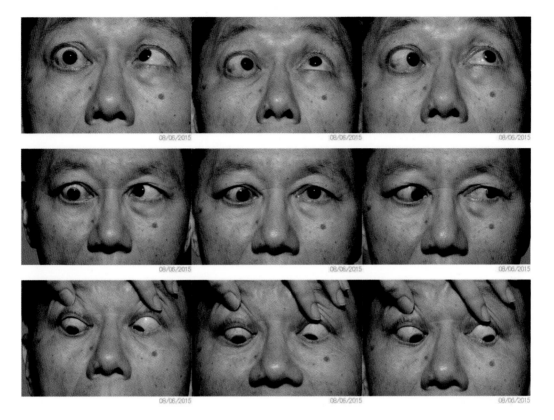

Figure 6.17 The most common etiology for unilateral proptosis is thyroid eye disease. It is important to determine the activity and severity in such patients. This patient has thyroid eye disease with unilateral proptosis which is of moderate severity and is currently inactive.

Note: Watch out for contralateral ptosis as myasthenia can occur concurrently with 15–20% of patients with thyroid eye disease.

of proptosis as there is **protrusion of the right corneal apex beyond the superior orbital rim**. I will measure with a **Hertel's exophthalmometer**. I feel/do not feel any associated neck masses that moves with swallowing and the cervical lymph nodes are not palpable. I will assess the **optic nerve function** by checking the visual acuity, relative afferent pupillary defect, and confrontational visual fields. I will also check the pupils for anisocoria.

Examination of the **extraocular movements** shows abduction, elevation, and adduction deficit in the right eye. Movements in the left eye are full. The patient also has lid lag on downgaze as well. I will palpate to look for resistance **to retropulsion as well as thrill and auscultate for bruit; check for lagophthalmos and Bell's reflex; check the corneal sensation; and perform a Valsalva maneuver**. I will check under the slit lamp looking at the **anterior segment** for injection; stain with fluorescein for epithelial defects, chemosis, **cockscrew vessels**, superior limbic keratitis, evidence of exposure keratopathy, and caruncular inflammation; check the intraocular pressure in straight gaze and upgaze; check the lens status; and perform a **dilated fundal examination** for optic disc swelling, pallor, increased cup-disc ratio, optociliary shunt, and choroidal folds. I will examine for associated palmar erythema, atrial fibrillation, and pretibial myxedema.

In summary, this patient has a unilateral axial proptosis. My differentials include **thyroid eye disease, which is the most common condition, and which is inactive and of at least moderate severity**. Other differentials include orbital tumors such as lymphoma or metastatic disease, benign lesions such as cavernous hemangioma, schwannoma (both schwannoma and cavernous hemangioma are less likely causes in this patient as they will present with axial proptosis) or meningioma (rarer in males). Inflammatory causes include orbital inflammatory disease as well as Wegener's syndrome and vascular causes include carotid cavernous fistula or varix.

Q **Question 18 Viva Stem: How would you Perform a Lateral Tarsorrhaphy?**

I will perform the procedure under informed consent and in aseptic conditions, and inject local anesthesia along the eyelids. Using a Bard Parker 15 blade, I will **split the anterior and posterior lamellae** along the gray line in the lateral portion of both the upper and lower eyelids to a **depth of 2 mm, extending the split medially for 5 mm/to a length as required (using a blade or spring scissors)**. I will excise **1 mm of the lid margin and posterior lamella**. Using **6-0 vicryl** sutures, I will start with the upper lid first, entering the posterior lamella laterally and passing the suture through partial thickness, exiting medially from the posterior lamella. I will then pass the needle into the posterior lamella of the lower lid, ensuring the **entry and exit points are in line** with the upper lid. I will then close the anterior lamella with 6/o prolene sutures with **silicone bolsters**, placing a **mattress suture** by entering the skin of the upper lid **2–3 mm away from the lid margin** and exiting at the anterior lamella before passing through the anterior lamella of the lower lid and exiting at the skin 2–3 mm inferior to the lid margin. I will repeat the steps till desired closure is achieved, ensuring that the **lashes are everted**. I will place two to three mattress sutures **3 mm apart** till the **skin is closed over the posterior lamella**.

CHAPTER 7

PEDIATRICS

Q **Question 1.1 Viva Stem: Cover-Uncover Test showing Alternating Exotropia.**

On examination of this patient, there is no abnormal head posture, no ptosis, and eyes are straight on primary gaze on Hirschberg light reflex.

I will say to the patient, "Sir do you wear glasses for distance? Please put on the glasses. Can you see the cross with your right eye? Can you see the cross with your left eye?"

On covering of the patient's right eye, the left eye **moves inward to take up fixation**. Under cover, there is no **dissociated vertical deviation or latent nystagmus**. On uncovering the right eye, the left eye maintains fixation. On covering the left eye, the right eye moves in to take up fixation. Under the cover, there is no dissociated vertical deviation or latent nystagmus. On uncovering the left eye, the right eye maintains fixation. This confirms an **alternating exotropia**. On alternate cover test, both eyes move in to take up fixation. I will perform a cover-uncover test with and without glasses for distance and near vision with prisms, and check extraocular movements for limitation, **A or V pattern**, and **inferior oblique overaction**. I will check the visual acuity and relative afferent pupillary defect; perform a **cycloplegic refraction** for children and a normal refraction for adults; check the **stereopsis** for distance and near vision; examine the anterior chamber for any lesions that might affect vision such as corneal scars, any previous squint operations, and intraocular pressure; perform a dilated fundal examination for cup-disc ratio, optic disc swelling or pallor, and any macula lesions; and perform a family album tomography scan.

Note: for childhood strabismus, always offer to check visual acuity, relative afferent pupillary defect, intraocular pressure, cycloplegic refraction stereopsis for near and far distance, and extraocular movements.

Q **Question 1.2 What are the Indications for Surgery in Alternating Exotropia?**

The indications are **increasing frequency of breakdown more than 50% of the time, increasing angle, worsening stereopsis, abnormal head posture,** and **severe asthenopia** (from overaccommodation to bring eyes in).

> **Q** **Question 1.3** Examination of a Patient reveals the following: Distance Deviation is 40 Diopters, and Near Deviation is 20 diopters. How would you manage such a Patient?

I will first perform **prolonged patching of more than 30 min (bad eye)** before performing an alternate cover test to assess for **tenacious proximal fusion**. If that fails, I will then perform a **+3 diopter sphere test**. If the difference is ≥ **10 PD**, the patient has **true divergence excess**. As the angle of deviation is moderately large, the patient will need two muscle surgeries. I will recess the lateral rectus bilaterally, aiming for a correction of the average of distance and near deviation (to avoid consecutive high AC/A ratio for Esotropia).

Note: In all strabismus, keep at the back of the mind iatrogenic causes e.g. scleral buckle from a retinal detachment operation or tube implant in glaucoma surgery. Also note that patching breaks fusion; 3D+ lens breaks accommodation.

> **Q** **Question 2.1** Viva Stem: One-year-old Child presents with Left Eye In-Turning

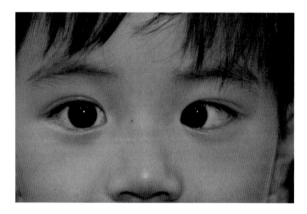

Figure 7.1 Left congenital esotropia.

This is the facial photograph of the patient showing inward deviation of the left eye. The right eye appears straight as noted by the central Hirschberg light reflex. Otherwise there is **no obvious proptosis, no ptosis, and no abnormal head posture**. I will examine the patient's history for duration of onset, progression, frequency of breakdown, precipitating events (e.g. illness or fatigue), whether the patient can fix, follow, and recognize faces, general development of the child, his birth history and whether there was any maternal infections, and any birth trauma or prematurity. I will also ask for any family history of eye disease and squints. I will examine the vision with age-appropriate methods, check the relative afferent pupillary defect, extraocular movements looking for limitation, A and V patterns as well as **inferior oblique overaction**, cover-uncover test as well as alternate cover test for distance and near vision with prisms, and look for **latent nystagmus** (stereopsis in older children). I will also examine the anterior segment for causes of sensory esotropia and presence of surgical scars, check the intraocular pressure and cycloplegic refraction, and perform a dilated fundal examination for causes of sensory squint. This patient is likely to have congenital esotropia.

Age-appropriate visual acuity:

- < 1 year old: central steady maintain, fix and follow, objection to occlusion, forced preferential looking (teller acuity), Catford drum, 100s and 1000s
- 1 to 3 years old: kay/allen's picture, Sheridan gardner
- > 3 years old: HOTV, Snellen's

Q **Question 2.2 What are the Causes of Esotropia in a Child?**

Most importantly, I will exclude **life-threatening causes such as sixth nerve palsy** as well as **sensory esotropia such as retinoblastoma or retinopathy of prematurity**. Other causes can be divided into congenital and acquired causes. Congenital cases occurring **before six months of age includes infantile esotropia, early accommodative type, Duane syndrome, Mobius syndrome**, and **nystagmus blockade syndrome**. Acquired causes can be divided into comitant and incomitant causes. **Comitant causes include accommodative esotropia, late onset non-accommodative, cyclical, consecutive**, or **stress-induced. Incomitant forms include thyroid eye disease, trauma**, and **myasthenia**.

Q **Question 2.3 What are the Features of Congenital Esotropia?**

Features include **large angle, stable deviation**, and **equal for near and distance vision**. Other features include **cross-fixation, amblyopia, suppression, poor stereopsis, latent nystagmus, inferior oblique overaction**, and **asymmetrical optokinetic response**.

Q **Question 2.4 How would you Manage a Patient who was measured to have 40 Diopters of Deviation for Distance and Near Vision, and Visual Acuity of OD 6/30 OS 6/30, +1D OU?**

This patient likely has congenital esotropia. Treatment is dependent on size of the angle, progression, associated amblyopia, and motility defects such as inferior oblique overaction dissociated vertical deviation V or A pattern (age of onset and difference between distance and near and refractive error are important but they are already provided in the stem). The aim of the treatment is to restore **binocular single vision** and **normal ocular alignment**.

I will first treat the amblyopia by patching till equal fixation preference is achieved, ensuring **stable refraction and angle of deviation over two visits three to four weeks apart**. I will explain to the parents the guarded prognosis due to amblyopia and poor stereopsis. As the patient is above six months old, the patient will need surgical intervention soon **(before the age of two) to maximize stereopsis** potential, and this patient will require two muscle surgeries. If there is no amblyopia, then bilateral medial rectus recession can be performed. If there is persistent amblyopia in the left eye and the angle deviation is large, I will perform recession of the medial rectus and resection of the ipsilateral lateral rectus. I will explain to the parents the **end point of monofixation, that amblyopia might persist,** the risk of **overcorrection or undercorrection, and manifestation of other deviations such as dissociated vertical deviation and inferior oblique overaction** which might require a **second operation**.

Note: Issues with recess and resection in the same eye include increase in incomitance and globe retraction. The advantage is that if there are intraoperative complications, only the affected eye is endangered.

Q **Question 3.1 Viva Stem: Describe the Photo in Figure 7.2 of a 29-week Gestational-age Baby.**

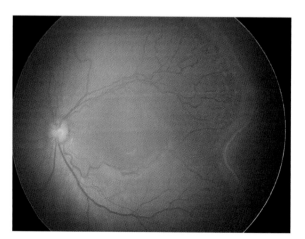

Figure 7.2 This fundal photo of a premature baby shows the presence of stage 3 Retinopathy of Prematurity in Zone 1. When approaching the topic of Retinopathy of Prematurity, it is important to assess the zone, stage and number of clock hours and tailor the management accordingly.

Note: Do not offer to check the visual acuity of a premature baby.

This is the fundal photograph of the left eye. The vitreous is **slightly hazy** in keeping with the age of the baby. Temporally extending from **12 o' clock to 5 o'clock position**, there is a **raised ridge** at the junction between **zone 1 and zone 2** with **fibrovascular proliferation** that appears to **extend into the extraretinal space**. The retina temporal to the ridge appears **avascular**. The patient also has features of **Plus disease** as evidenced by at least two quadrants of arteriolar tortuosity and venodilation. The cup-disc ratio is 0.5, the disc is not dragged, and the retina appears flat. I will checking for relative afferent papillary defect, examine the **peripheries with indentation**, and check the **fellow eye**. I will examine the mother's history for the gestational age at birth, any complications during childbirth, whether there was any intensive care unit stay, use of supplemental oxygen, and other medical complications such as intraventricular hemorrhage, necrotizing enterocolitis, and respiratory distress syndrome. This patient has threshold disease of retinopathy of prematurity.

Q **Question 3.2 When will you Screen for Retinopathy of Prematurity?**

In my center, we screen premature babies who are below 32 weeks of gestational age and below 1.5 kg, especially those who are **unwell with conditions such as necrotizing enterocolitis, intraventricular hemorrhage**, and **respiratory distress syndrome**, and **those who have had intensive care unit stay with intubation**. We start screening at 31 weeks of gestational age or four weeks after birth, whichever is later.

Q **Question 3.3 How will you Manage this baby who has Retinopathy of Prematurity?**

This baby has retinopathy of prematurity fulfilling the threshold criteria which has a poor prognosis and is an indication to start retinal photocoagulation. I will co-manage the patient with the pediatrician. I will counsel the parents regarding the indications for retinal photocoagulation, side effects, and alternatives, including **intravitreal anti-vascular endothelial growth factors** or observation. I will explain that without treatment, 50% deteriorate with severe visual loss while 20% still progress despite adequate treatment.

Q **Question 3.4 How will you Perform a Laser Procedure for a Patient with Retinopathy of Prematurity and What are the Risks?**

I will perform retinal photocoagulation for the patient under informed consent from the parents in the operating theater under general anesthesia. I will dilate the eyes using cyclomydril and insert a **pediatric lid speculum**, examine under anesthesia using the indirect opthalmoscope with 360 degress indentation using a 20 diopter lens. I will then apply laser using an **indirect laser using the 20 diopter lens with a setting of 200 mW 200 ms 200 microns** titrating to get a **grey white burn**. I will **apply laser to the avascular area anterior to the ridge** spacing my **shots 0.5 spot size apart**. I will then **review in one to two weeks** and top up the laser if the disease remains active. Risks of the procedure can be divided into anesthetic risk and procedural risk. Anesthetic risks from the general anesthesia include **hypotension, myocardial infarction, and sudden death especially in babies who are unwell**. Risks of the procedure include **fovea or iris burns, myopia, strabismus, amblyopia, constricted visual field, cataracts, and retinal detachment.**

> **Q** **Question 3.5 How will you Manage a Dragged Disc which develops with associated Retinal Detachment?**

The presence of a dragged disc is a poor prognostic sign and is difficult to treat. I will emphasize the guarded prognosis to the parents, explaining to them that the patient requires surgery and the main indications are to maximize vision and prevent phthisis. I will first attempt a scleral buckling, failing which I will consider pars plana vitrectomy.

Note: It is difficult to enforce proper posturing in a child if a tear develops and vitreous substitutes are required.

> **Q** **Question 4.1 OSCE Stem: Examination of a Patient with Fundus Findings shown in Figures 7.3A and 7.3B.**

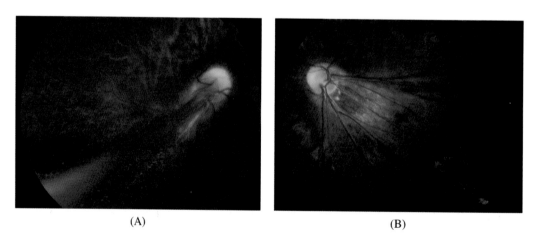

(A)   (B)

Figures 7.3A and 7.3B   The photos demonstrate the presence of bilateral dragged disc secondary to retinopathy of prematurity. There is presence of a fibrovascular membrane in the right eye. The fundus are tessellated, suggestive of myopia which is a common complication of retinopathy of prematurity.

On general examination, both eyes appear deviated temporally. There is presence of a conjugate binocular horizontal pendular nystagmus. On examination of the patient's right fundus, there is **dragging of the disc temporally by fibrovascular tissues extending anteriorly and obstructing the view of the macula. It is associated with straightening of the arcades.** There are no new vessels at the disc or elsewhere and the posterior pole is flat. The disc is pale and the cup-disc ratio is difficult to assess. Peripherally there are areas of panretinal photocoagulation scars but no retinal detachment nor granuloma. Examination of the left fundus reveals similar findings with temporal dragging of the disc by fibrovascular membranes with straightening of the arcades. The macula is ectopically located inferotemporally. Examination of the peripheries reveals similar findings to the right eye. This patient has **bilateral dragged disc likely secondary to proliferative retinopathy status post-panretinal photocoagulation.** I will check the visual acuity, relative afferent pupillary defect, cycloplegic refraction, and intraocular pressure, check the anterior segment for rubeosis and cataract, and ask for a history of prematurity or family history of ocular disease and contact with dogs (toxocariasis).

Q Question 4.2 How would you Treat the Patient in Question 4.1?

Management can be divided into **systemic** and **ocular.** I will inform the parents of the **guarded visual prognosis.** In the acute phase, I will co-manage the patient with the **internist/pediatrician** systemically and treat the underlying cause. The most likely cause would be retinopathy of prematurity. I will perform **retinal photocoagulation to areas of ischemia.** If retinal detachment develops, I will refer to the vitreoretinal surgeon to consider **sclera buckle surgery,** failing which **pars plana vitrectomy** will be required. I will monitor the patient long-term for complications of neovascular glaucoma, cataracts, myopia, strabismus, and amblyopia, and treat accordingly.

Q Question 5.1 Viva Stem: How do you Perform a Resection Surgery?

I will perform a resection surgery under informed parental consent (assuming the patient is a child) under general anesthesia in the operating theater in sterile conditions. I will perform a limited limbal or forniceal conjunctival peritomy, dissecting the Tenon's, hooking the rectus muscle first using a **Stevens hook,** followed by a **Jameson hook,** and spreading over a **Chavasse hook** followed by clearing of the ligaments and fascial sheath with a cotton bud. I will tag the muscle with **6/o double-armed vicryl** at the required resection length measured using calipers with **interlocking** sutures **dividing the muscle into thirds,** cut the rectus muscle anterior to the suture, and clamp the sutures with a bulldog clamp. I will then excise the excess rectus muscle 1 mm from the insertion leaving behind a rectus stump, following which I will anchor the 6/o vicryl to the rectus stump and close the conjunctiva with **8/0 vicryl**. I will then start the patient on analgesia and topical antibiotics and steroids in the absence of contraindications.

> **Q** **Question 5.2** How will you Manage if, during Squint Surgery, you noticed Sudden Softening of the Eye while Anchoring the Rectus Muscle to the Sclera?

There is likely a **scleral perforation** secondary to full thickness entry of the suture needle. I will stop the surgery and examine the eye, **looking for vitreous at the entry wound**. I will perform an on-table dilated fundal examination, looking for retinal breaks and detachment. If identified, I will perform an **indirect laser retinopexy** and **subsequently complete the surgery expediently, referring to the vitreoretinal surgeon immediately after operation**.

> **Q** **Question 6.1** OSCE Stem: Examination of a Patient with Extraocular Movement Shown in Figure 7.4.

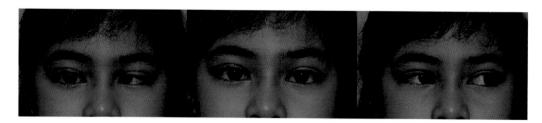

Figure 7.4 This patient has right type 1 Duane's syndrome. On primary gaze her eyes are straight. There is absent abduction in the right eye with associated narrowing of the palpebral aperture on left gaze. She does not have features suggestive of Leash phenomenon.

On primary gaze, the eyes are straight using the Hirchsberg reflex. There is no abnormal head posture and no ptosis. On right gaze, there is limitation of the right eye. On testing of ductions, there is limitation of right eye abduction. On left gaze, eye movements are full but there is **narrowing of the palpebral aperture with retraction of the globe in the right eye** with no associated **upshoot or downshoot**. On upgaze and downgaze, eye movements are full; up and left as well as down and left eye movements are full with narrowing of the right globe retraction. On upgaze and right gaze as well as downgaze and right gaze, there is limitation in the right eye. On general inspection, there is absence of limbal dermoids and lid colobomas. I will check the visual acuity, examine the eye for **iris coloboma, foveal as well as optic nerve head hypoplasia, and remnant hyaloid artery,** check systemically for **preauricular skin tags, urinary tract agenesis and bone abnormalities, examine the patient's history for seizures, deafness, as well as café au lait spots** and **Wildervanck syndrome (Klippel-Feil fusion of cervical vertebrae with Duane's syndrome and deafness)**. In summary, this patient has right type 1 Duane's syndrome.

Q Question 6.2 How would you Manage this Patient (Patient in Figure 7.4)?

Management can be divided into systemic and ocular. I will work with the internist to manage associated systemic associations. Ocular management depends on **presence of abnormal head posture, excessive leash phenomenon** or **narrowing of the palpebral aperture** and **ocular deviation in primary gaze**. As the patient does not have any of these, I will monitor the patient. I will treat any associated amblyopia with patching and full spectacle correction. If surgical intervention is required, I will perform **recession surgery** with or without transposition. If there is significant Leash phenomenon, **Y splitting of the lateral rectus** would be required.

Note: Never perform resection surgery in an already tight eye in Duane's syndrome.

Q Question 7.1 Viva Stem: How do you Manage a Six-Month-Old Child presenting with Persistent Tearing?

In a young child presenting with tearing, I will need to exclude **life-threatening conditions such as masquerade** and sight-threatening causes such as **congenital glaucoma** (triad of epiphora, blepharospasm, and photophobia), **infective keratitis**, or **uveitis**. Other conditions include **epiblepharon, conjunctivitis, corneal abrasion**, and **congenital nasolacrimal duct obstruction**. I will examine the patient's history for duration of tearing, progression, age of onset, any associated photophobia or blepharospasm, any trauma, presence of discharge, presence of squint, and whether the child is able to recognize faces and fixate. I will examine the child's birth history as well as family history of ocular disease (e.g. uveitis and glaucoma).

I will check the visual acuity by age-appropriate method, presence of relative afferent pupillary defect, and cycloplegic refraction (myopic in glaucoma); look at the lids for epiblepharon and medial canthal swelling; examine under sedation for corneal lash touch, injection, and follicles, as well as note the tear lake height; and perform compression on the lacrimal sac looking for mucopurulent reflux. I will examine the cornea, noting the diameter and clarity/striae, check the sclera for bluish hue, stain for epithelial defects, check the intraocular pressure using the Icare tonometer, check the anterior chamber for activity, rubeosis, and lens status. I will perform a dilated fundal examination for increased cup-disc ratio and secondary causes of glaucoma. If there is no view, I will perform a **B scan for tumors or retinal detachment**. I will investigate by performing an A scan to determine the **axial length if the clinical suspicion is congenital glaucoma**. I will perform a **dye disappearance test if I suspect nasolacrimal duct obstruction**.

Q **Question 7.2 What are the Symptoms of Congenital Glaucoma?**

The classical symptoms of congenital glaucoma are **blepharospasm, epiphora, and photophobia** (triad).

Q **Question 7.3A1 Scenario 1 — All Other Tests are Normal; Patient presents one week later with Discharge, Pain and Fever. Please describe Figure 7.5.**

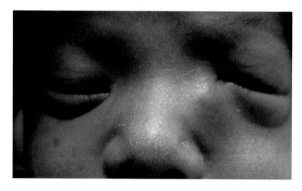

Figure 7.5 Left dacryocystitis secondary to congenital nasolacrimal duct obstruction in a young child with mild surrounding preseptal cellulitis.

This is the partial facial photograph of the child showing a **left medial canthal angle swelling** with surrounding erythema which is non-pointing. There is surrounding **periorbital swelling** but no obvious proptosis. I will check the visual acuity by age-appropriate method, **extraocular movements, relative afferent papillary defect**, intraocular pressures, the anterior segment for chemosis and injection that might suggest orbital cellulitis, and perform a dilated fundal examination. Systemically I will check the vitals for fever. This patient has **left dacryocystitis secondary to congenital nasolacrimal duct obstruction** with **possible periorbital cellulitis**.

Differentials to nasal mass in a child:

Dacryocystitis or dacryocele (below medial canthal tendon)
Encephalocele (above medial canthal tendon)
Dermoid
Capillary hemangioma
Lymphangioma
Arteriovenous malformation
Neuroblastsoma
Ewing's sarcoma

Q Question 7.3A2 How would you Manage this Patient?

This is a potentially life-threatening and sight-threatening condition. I will need to treat the infection, monitor for progression, and treat the underlying cause. I will **admit the patient and co-manage the patient with the pediatrician**, monitoring the vitals and relative afferent papillary defect closely, and starting the patient on **systemic intravenous broad spectrum antibiotics** in the absence of contraindications. I will investigate by checking the full blood count, erythrocyte sedimentation rate, and C-reactive protein and **blood cultures** (keep in view wound swab if it is discharging). If the clinical suspicion for orbital cellulitis is high, I will perform a magnetic resonance imaging of the orbits and refer the patient to the otolaryngologist. I will monitor daily and treat any associated complications (e.g. raised intraocular pressure or exposure from proptosis). If the swelling is very tense, an **incision** and **drainge** or **needle aspiration** might be required under general anesthesia but carries a risk of fistula formation.

Once the acute infection has settled, I will discuss with the parents early definitive surgical intervention versus conservative management, explaining that there is **higher rate of failure** with conservative management in view of the previous infection. Conservative management includes **Crigler massage** and topical **prophylactic antibiotic drops**. Surgical intervention involves first examination under anesthesia with **syringing** and **probing**, failing which the child will need **stenting** (three–six months) or **balloon dacryoplasty**. If that fails, the patient will need **definitive dacryocystorhinostomy**.

Note: Crigler massage can still be offered for this scenario as the patient is under one-year old.

Q Question 7.3A3 How would you Advise Parents to Perform a Lacrimal Massage?

I will advise parents to perform the **Crigler lacrimal sac massage** by pressing **medial to the medial canthal angle, sweeping inferiorly** using the little finger in **both directions, ten strokes repeated four times a day**.

Q **Question 7.3A4** How would you Perform Syringing, and Syringing and Probing?

I will perform the procedure under informed parental consent, under general anesthesia in the operating theater. I will first **dilate the upper punctum with Nettleship punctal dilator**, perform syringing of the upper and lower punctum to confirm blockage, followed by insertion of a **00 (Two 0) Bowman probe** into the upper canaliculus with lateral distraction of the lids (to straighten the canaliculus) and pass it medially till I feel a **hard stop**. I will then turn it **vertically and pass it inferiorly, laterally and posteriorly** till I feel a give or a **"pop" sound** is achieved, and insert another metal probe along the floor of the nose to feel for **metal-to-metal contact**. I will then **reconfirm with syringing with fluorescein dye** and **inserting an aspiration tube into the nose to look for dye retrieval**.

Note in general the following: Below one year old — perform lacrimal massage. About one year old — perform probing which can be repeated twice if required. One to three years old — infracture of inferior turbinate, balloon dacryoplasty, or stenting with temporary Crawford tube. Above three years old — dacryocystorhinostomy.

Q **Question 7.3B1** Scenario 2 — Cornea is Hazy with Increased Corneal Diameter Measuring 14 mm, with an Intraocular Pressure of 40. What are the Possible Causes and how would you Complete the Examination?

This patient has congenital glaucoma. This is a sight-threatening condition which is difficult to treat and carries a poor prognosis. Causes can be divided into primary and secondary. Primary cause is likely **congenital glaucoma** in this patient. (Do not mention **Juvenile Open Angle Glaucoma** as the age group is different). Secondary causes include **chromosomal disorders** (trisomy 21); **metabolic disorders** (Lowe syndrome, Zellweger syndrome); **phakomatoses** (neurofibromatosis, Sturge-Weber disease); and **anterior segment abnormalities** like nanophthalmos, congenital ectropion uvea, aniridia, Peter's anomaly, and anterior segment dysgenesis. **Acquired causes include post-trauma, uveitis**, and **tumors**, as well as **steroid-induced** and **chronic retinal detachments**. I will check the cycloplegic refraction; measure the axial length and check the cup-disc ratio; and examine under general anesthesia with informed parental consent, informing the anesthetist to **use ketamine** and **avoid other intravenous or inhalational anesthesia** (which artificially reduces intraocular pressure). I will recheck the intraocular pressure using the Icare tonometer/Tono-pen and perform a direct gonioscopy using the Koeppe lens.

	Expected Axial Length (mm)	Corneal Diameter (Abnormally Large) (mm)
Birth	16–17	9.5–10.5 (≥ 11)
One year old	19–20	10–11.5 (≥ 12)
Two years old		12 (≥ 13)

Q Question 7.3B2 How would you Treat the Patient in Question 7.3B1 above?

Pediatric glaucoma is a **blinding condition** which is **difficult to treat** and carries a **poor prognosis**. Factors to consider include the **visual prognosis**, vision of contralateral eye, underlying cause, **corneal clarity**, and **age of the patient**. Management can be divided into **systemic** and **ocular**. Systemically, I will co-manage the patient with the pediatrician to exclude systemic associations and complications. Ocular-wise, I will need to treat the glaucoma as well as associated ocular complications such as amblyopia, cornea scarring, and strabismus. Medical therapy for glaucoma is a temporizing measure (beta blockers, carbonic anhydrase inhibitors, or prostaglandin analogues), and the patient will need definitive surgical treatment. In this patient, with a hazy cornea and diameter of 14 mm, I will consider performing an **angle surgery (trabeculotomy)**, failing which it can be repeated a second time before considering **glaucoma filtration surgery** or **glaucoma drainage device implantation**. If the visual prognosis is poor, then **transscleral cyclophotocoagulation** can be considered.

> **Surgical Management**
> Angle surgery
> - Conjunctival-sparing, i.e. goniotomy but requires a clear cornea
> - Conjunctival involving, i.e. trabeculotomy which does not require clear cornea
>
> Second-line surgery
> - Glaucoma filtration surgery, i.e. trabeculectomy or glaucoma drainage device implantation, i.e. tube
> - If prognosis is poor, transscleral cyclophotocoagulation should be considered

Note: A trabeculotomy is usually performed inferiorly so that the superior conjunctiva can be spared for a future trabeculectomy if required.

Q Question 8 Viva Stem: What is your Approach to Treating a 3-year-old Child presenting with White Eye and Hypopyon?

In a young child presenting with hypopyon, I will need to **exclude life-threatening and sight-threatening causes**. Causes of hypopyon can be divided into **inflammatory** and **infective** causes, which can be further classified into **granulomatous** and **non-granulomatous**, as well as **masquerade**. Life-threatening, masquerade causes in a young child include intraocular tumors such as **retinoblastoma** (but less likely since retinoblastoma usually develops before two years old) and **leukemia**, while sight-threatening causes include **chronic retinal detachment** from causes such as retinopathy of prematurity and Coat's disease or trauma.

Inflammatory causes include juvenile rheumatoid arthritis, especially the pauciarticular form (need to know the four forms of juvenile rheumatoid arthritis), as well as tubular interstitial nephritis and uveitis. **Infective** causes include herpes viruses, toxocariasis, syphilis, and toxoplasmosis. I will examine the patient's history of duration and onset, examine the visual acuity by age-appropriate method, check the relative afferent pupillary defect and the red reflex, and examine the extraocular movements for limitation as well as nystagmus and strabismus.

I will examine the anterior segment for keratic precipitates, band keratopathy, posterior and peripheral anterior synechiae, iris nodules, and anterior chamber activity; check the intraocular pressure using the Icare or Perkins tonometer; and check the lens status for cataracts. I will perform a dilated fundal examination for evidence of retinoblastoma, retinal detachments, granulomas, or areas of retinitis or choroiditis. If retinoblastoma is suspected, I will examine under anesthesia with 360 degrees indentation, bone marrow biopsy, and lumbar puncture as well as magnetic resonance imaging of the brain looking for calcification, spread, ectopic retinoblastoma or pineoblastoma. I will also examine the family members. Treatment can be divided into **systemic** and **ocular** treatments which are dependent on the **underlying cause** and **visual prognosis**.

Infants	Toddlers/School Children	Adolescents
• Herpes simplex virus	• Toxocariasis	• Juvenile rheumatoid arthritis
• Toxocarasis	• Toxoplasmosis	• Pars planitis
• Retinoblastoma	• Leukemia	• Vogt-Koyanagi-Harada disease
	• Vogt-Koyanagi-Harada disease	• Toxoplasmosis
	• Juvenile rheumatoid arthritis	• HLA-B27-associated sarcoidosis
		• Behçet's disease
		• Intraocular foreign bodies

Juvenile Rheumatoid Arthritis (RF −ve)	Systemic	Ocular	
Joints		Poly	Pauci < 4
Antinuclear antibody	−	−	−	+
HLA-B27	−	−	+	−
	Still's disease	Male late	Female Early
		Type 2	Type 1

Q **Question 9.1 Viva Stem: 7-Year-old Girl Presents with Poor Vision, Otherwise Asymptomatic. Please describe the photograph.**

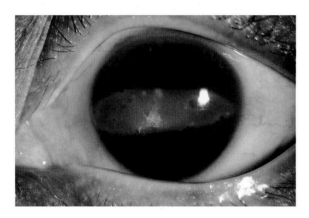

Figure 7.6 Left band keratopathy in a young girl with juvenile rheumatoid arthritis. She developed cataracts and subsequently underwent lens aspiration. She was left aphakic with contact lens refractive correction.

This is the anterior segment photo of the patient's left eye, showing dense band keratopathy with **a Swiss cheese appearance in the interpalpebral region** extending from 3 to 9 o'clock involving the visual axis. The patient is **aphakic** as well. Otherwise the conjunctiva is not injected, there are neither obvious keratic precipitates nor anterior synechiae, and the eye does not appear buphthalmic (to exclude congenital glaucoma as a cause of band keratopathy). I will check the visual acuity, relative afferent pupillary defect, and red reflex; examine the patient under the slit lamp for **peripheral anterior and posterior synechiae**, **iris nodules**, **keratic precipitates**, and **anterior chamber activity**; check the intraocular pressure; perform a dilated fundal examination; and examine the fellow eye.

I will examine systemically looking for **joint swelling**, **erythema**, or **deformities**. I will examine the patient's history for duration of symptoms, progression, age of onset, any ocular pain, any trauma, any systemic associations such as **joint pain**, **fever**, **weight loss**, **rash**, and **renal disease**. I will also examine the patient's birth history (whether there was prematurity or any infections) and past medical history as well as family history. Differentials include (1) uveitis such as juvenile rheumatoid arthritis with cataract development requiring lens aspiration, (2) previous congenital cataract status post-lens aspiration with subsequent complication of aphakic glaucoma, (3) chronic retinal detachment, and (4) congenital glaucoma (less likely as eye is buphthalmic).

Note: Offer differentials in order of likelihood.

Causes of Band Keratopathy

1. Ocular: chronic anterior uveitis (particularly in children), phthisis bulbi, silicone oil in the anterior chamber, chronic corneal edema and severe chronic keratitis, glaucoma
2. Age-related (affects otherwise healthy individuals)
3. Metabolic (metastatic calcification): this is rare and includes increased serum calcium and phosphorus, hyperuricemia, and chronic renal failure
4. Hereditary causes including familial cases and ichthyosis

Q Question 9.2 Anterior Chamber Shows 1+ Cells with some Fine Keratic Precipitates in Both Eyes, some Areas of Posterior Synechiae in the Fellow Eye, and Intraocular Pressure Normal Bilaterally. What is your impression?

This patient likely has **bilateral uveitis**, most commonly **juvenile rheumatoid arthritis**. I will like to co-manage the patient with the pediatrician and investigate the patient, looking for an underlying cause. I will check the **full blood count for raised white cells, erythrocyte sedimentation rate, and C-reactive protein; check for rheumatoid factor, antinuclear antibodies**, and **HLA B27 gene**, and perform a **Mantoux chest X-ray** and **syphilis screen**. I will also perform a **steroid workup** for the patient.

Q Question 9.3 What are the Blinding Complications of Juvenile Rheumatoid Arthritis?

Blinding complications of juvenile rheumatoid arthritis include **band keratopathy, cataract, glaucoma, cystoid macular edema**, and **amblyopia**.

Note: Risk factor for uveitis in juvenile idiopathic arthritis: negative rheumatoid factor, positive antinuclear antibodies, female, pauciarticular form.

Q Question 9.4 How would you Manage Juvenile Rheumatoid Arthritis?

Management can be divided into systemic and ocular. Systemically, I will co-manage the patient with the pediatrician and start the patient on **systemic immunosuppressant therapy** in the absence of contraindications and treat any joint deformities. Ocular management will include **treatment of inflammation** as well as **treatment** and **monitoring of complications**. I will start the patient on **topical preservative-free steroids** with **antibiotic cover** and **cycloplegics** in the absence of contraindications. I will monitor for the development of **glaucoma** and **amblyopia** in both eyes and **cataract** in the fellow eye. As this patient is near the age of full visual maturity, I will need to aggressively control the inflammation and perform **chelation** and **superficial keratectomy** of the **band keratopathy** with **ethylene diamine tetra-acetic acid 3% for 3 min** with consideration of future intraocular lens implantation (when intraocular inflammation is quiescent). I will treat the **amblyopia with patching as well as full refractive correction using rigid gas permeable lenses** (or aphakic glasses if both eyes are aphakic) and **treat any glaucoma** with topical anti-glaucoma medications, failing which the patient would require surgery such as a trabeculectomy with mitomycin C or glaucoma drainage device implantation.

Aphakia	
Surgical-related	**Non-surgical-related (zonulysis)**
Intracapsular cataract extraction, high myopia, retinal detuchment-silicone oil, pediatric cataract	Causes of ectopia lentis

Note: Cataract surgery for patient with juvenile rheumatoid arthritis: usually cataract surgery is performed one year after the disease is controlled, leaving the patient aphakic at the initial setting.

Q Question 9.5 What are the Causes of Uveitis in Children?

Causes of uveitis in children can be divided into infective and inflammatory, which can be subdivided into granulomatous and non-granulomatous, as well as masquerade, which can be further divided into life-threatening and sight-threatening causes. Life-threatening causes include malignancies like **retinoblastoma**, **secondaries**, or **leukemia**. Sight-threatening causes include chronic retinal detachment. Inflammatory granulomatous causes include Vogt-Koyanagi-Harada disease, sympathetic ophthalmia, and sarcoidosis. Non-granulomatous causes include juvenile rheumatoid arthritis, juvenile ankylosing spondylitis, juvenile reiter's disease, and juvenile inflammatory bowel disease as well as Behçet's. Infective granulomatous causes can be divided into viral such as Herpes virus, bacterial such as tuberculosis and syphilis as well as parasites such as toxocariasis and toxoplasmosis.

Note: Keep in mind that causes should be tailored to the age of presentation of the child in the question stem.

Q **Question 9.6** **If Systemic and Topical Steroids are Unable to Control the Inflammation, what Other Options are there?**

Other options include **subtenon's or periocular steroids as well as systemic steroid-sparing immunosuppressants**.

Q **Question 10.1** **Viva Stem: Parents brought in their 2-Year-old Child due to an Abnormal-looking Right Eye. Please describe the photo below.**

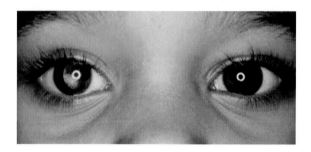

Figure 7.7 Right leukocoria in a young child.

This is the partial facial photo of the child, showing a right-sided **leukocoria**, with mild exotropia of the right eye **on Hirschberg light reflex**. The eye is **not injected**. I will **exclude life-threatening causes, most importantly retinoblastoma**. Other malignancies include medulloepithelioma and secondaries. Sight-threatening causes include **retinopathy of prematurity, causes of retinal detachment such as Coat's disease, familial exudative vitreoretinopathy, Norrie disease, retinal dysplasia**, and **incontinentia pigmenti** (mention only if the patient is female as males do not survive) as well as **infective causes such as toxocariasis**.

Other congenital causes include **congenital cataracts, persistent fetal vasculature, colobomas**, and **astrocytoma**. I will examine the patient's history of onset, progression, whether the patient can recognize faces or is able to fix and follow, whether there was any noticeable squint previously, any other medical problems, perinatal history, any history of infection during pregnancy, any trauma, birth weight and prematurity, and family history of eye disease or malignancies. I will examine the patient systemically looking for syndromic features; check the visual acuity by age-appropriate methods; check for relative afferent pupillary defect, extraocular movements, and proptosis; examine the anterior segment for inflammation, rubeosis, and cataracts; check the intraocular pressure, and perform a dilated fundal examination for retinal detachments, retinoblastoma, and vitreous seedings. If there is no view, I will perform a B scan to assess the status of the retina and presence of tumors. **(Retinoblastoma is acoustically solid, there is high internal reflectivity and presence of calcification)**

> **Q** **Question 10.2 Examination of the Fundus reveals the Lesion shown in Figure 7.8. Please describe the photo.**

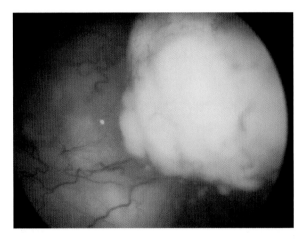

Figure 7.8 Large right retinoblastoma with a creamy white appearance and extensive exudative retinal detachment.

This is the fundal photo of the patient's right eye. It shows **a large creamy white endophytic lesion** with a **cottage cheese appearance** and **central calcification** arising around and obscuring the optic disc, involving the entire macula with surrounding retinal detachment with several small intraretinal satellite lesions inferiorly. The vitreous is clear with no evidence of **vitreous seeding**. This patient has right retinoblastoma (differential would be Coats disease). I will examine the rest of the fundus for other lesions and examine the fellow eye. I will examine the patient in the operating theater under **general anesthesia with 360 degrees indentation; perform a bone marrow biopsy (hematogenous spread)** and **lumbar puncture (central nervous system spread)** (looking for metastasis); and perform a **magnetic resonance imaging with contrast of the orbit and brain** looking for **calcifications, involvement of optic nerve, extraocular spread, and intracranial lesions** such as **ectopic retinoblastoma and pineoblastoma**.

Q Question 10.3 Describe the photo in Figure 7.9.

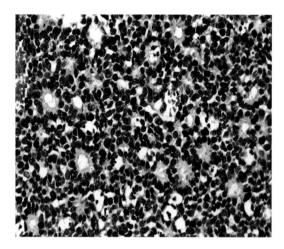

Figure 7.9 High-power microscopy showing Flexner Wintersteiner rosettes with well-formed lumina (H+ E, x 400 magnification).

This is the histopathology slide showing the presence of Flexner Wintersteiner (worst prognosis) with a single row of columnar cells surrounding an empty lumen with a reflective inner lining representing the external limiting membrane. There are cilia projecting into the lumen as well. The nucleus are large and hyperchromatic.

Q Question 10.4 How would you Differentiate Coats Disease from Retinoblastoma?

Retinoblastoma has calcifications, vitreous seeding, and potentially bilateral, discontinuous superficial vessels that dive in to supply inner tumor cells and less massive exudations. Coats disease has cholesterol crystals, does not have vitreous seedings, has continuous superficial telangiectatic vessels, usually unilateral and associated with massive exudation.

Q Question 10.5 How would you Manage this Patient (Patient in Figure 7.8)?

Retinoblastoma is a **life-threatening** and **sight-threatening condition**. Principles of management are to **first save life, then save the eye, and finally, maximize vision**. It will require a **multidisciplinary approach** involving a pediatric oncologist, a radiologist, and a geneticist, as well as an ocular prosthetist. Factors to consider can be divided into

patient and **ocular** factors. Patient factors include **fitness for surgery** or **treatment, evidence of systemic metastasis,** and **visual potential of the contralateral eye**. Ocular factors include **size, extent,** and **location,** as well as **presence of complications such as rubeosis, retinal detachment,** and **visual prognosis**.

In this patient with a large tumor with multiple small satellite lesions, management options can be divided into systemic, radiotherapy, and surgical. Local therapy such as **laser photocoagulation** and **cryotherapy (triple freeze thaw)** would not be suitable for this patient. Systemic options include systemic or **intra-arterial chemotherapy** as a **curative** treatment or as an **adjuvant chemoreduction therapy**. Radiotherapy options include **local plaque therapy** and **external beam radiation** (less commonly performed now). Surgical options include **enucleation indicated especially for large tumors, poor visual potential, presence of complications such as total retinal detachment, vitreous seeding,** or **rubeosis, and failure of other modalities**. I will also offer genetic counseling to the parents. I will follow up closely to monitor response to treatment and monitor the patient long term for development of other cancers.

Q **Question 10.6** **What are the Signs suggestive of Treatment Success using either Local or Systemic Therapy?**

Signs suggestive of successful treatment include **scarring of the lesion, decrease in size,** and **a chalky white fish-flesh appearance**.

Q **Question 11.1** **Viva Stem: What is a Hess Chart Test?**

A Hess chart is a dissimilar image test with binocular dissociation assessing the position of the fixating and non-fixating eye in all positions of gaze.

Q **Question 11.2** **What are the Fundamentals of a Hess Chart?**

A Hess chart is a **dissociated examination** based on **bifoveal projection,** and **obeying Hering's and Sherrington's law** with **normal retinal correspondence** and **lack of suppression**.

Q **Question 11.3** **What is Spread of Commitance?**

This is the **normalization of the underacting and overacting muscle**.

Q Question 11.4 What is Hering's Law and Sherrington's Law?

Hering's law is the **equal innervation of contralateral yolk muscles** while Sherrington's law is the **reciprocal innervation of ipsilateral antagonist muscles in binocular conjugate eye movements**.

Q Question 11.5 Describe the Hess Chart shown in Figure 7.10.

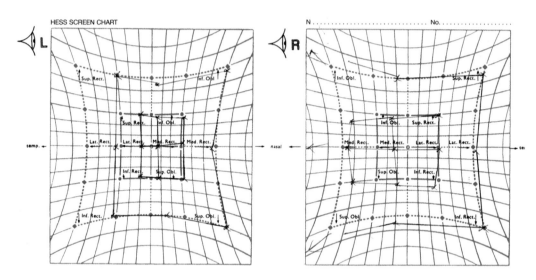

Figure 7.10   Hess chart of a patient with left paralytic sixth nerve palsy.

The Hess chart of the patient shows that the left field is **narrower than the right**, implying that the **left is the abnormal eye**. The left eye is **deviated medially on primary gaze** and there is **underaction of the lateral rectus** with **overaction of the ipsilateral medial rectus**. There is corresponding **overaction of the contralateral medial rectus** as well. This patient has **left lateral rectus weakness**, likely secondary to a right sixth nerve palsy. I will assess the optic nerve function by checking the visual acuity, relative afferent papillary defect, color vision, and confrontational visual field, direct visualization of the optic disc for disc swelling, examine the contiguous cranial nerves and extraocular movements, check the patient's history for the duration of onset, progression, trauma, vascular risk factors, and history of malignancy, and refer the patient to the otolaryngologist to exclude nasopharyngeal carcinoma (in a South Asian population).

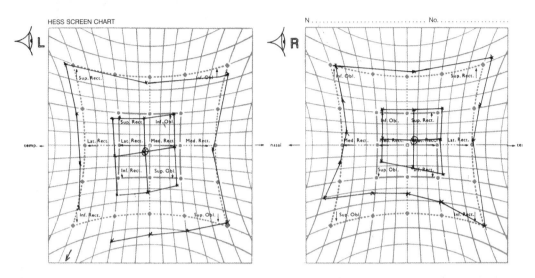

Figure 7.11 Hess chart of a patient with right fourth nerve palsy.

The Hess chart of the patient shows that the **right field is smaller than the left**, implying that the right is the abnormal eye. In the right field, the eye is slightly **deviated superiorly** and temporally in primary gaze with **underaction of the superior oblique** but without corresponding overaction of the inferior oblique (ipsilateral antagonist). In the left field, it is associated with **overaction of the inferior rectus** (contralateral yoke muscle). The superior oblique action of the left eye is intact (watch out for Hess charts with bilateral superior oblique palsy). This patient has right fourth nerve palsy. I will check the contiguous cranial nerves, check the extraocular movements, perform a cover-uncover and alternate cover test for distance and near vision with prisms and glasses, perform a Park's three-step test, check for increased vertical fusion range, perform a double Maddox rod test and a fundal examination for excyclotorsion, perform a family album tomography scan, and examine the patient's history for vascular risk factors and head trauma.

Q **Question 12.1** Viva Stem: Parents noted Inward Deviation of the Right Eye in their 1-month-old Child. What are the Possible Causes of such a Condition?

I will first exclude life-threatening and sight-threatening causes such as retinoblastoma, sixth nerve palsy, and sensory esotropia. Other causes include congenital esotropia, early-onset accommodative esotropia, nystagmus blockade syndrome, and Duane's syndrome.

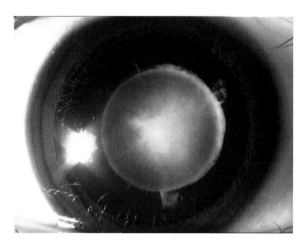

Figure 7.12 Right congenital lamellar cataract with riders.

This is the anterior segment photo of the right eye showing presence of a **lamellar cataract with associated riders,** and it is denser in the visual axis. The eye otherwise appears normal with a white conjunctiva and clear cornea. I will examine the fundus, check the **relative afferent papillary defect** (difficult to check visual acuity in a one-month-old child) and extraocular movements, examine the fellow eye, and perform cycloplegic refraction. This patient has **right unilateral congenital cataract with a sensory esotropia**. I will examine the patient's history for duration of esotropia and progression, birth history, any maternal infections, history of prematurity, and family history of ocular disease and cataracts.

Q **Question 12.3 How would you Treat the Child in Question 12.2?**

Congenital cataract is a **difficult condition to treat**. I will co-manage the patient with the pediatrician and investigate the systemic causes. For this patient, **in the presence of sensory esotropia**, he will need cataract removal. At this age, I will perform **lens aspiration with posterior capsulotomy and anterior vitrectomy without implanting an intraocular lens, suturing all wounds at the end of operation with 10/0 nylon**. Postoperatively, I will treat the amblyopia with **patching** and **contact lens** with slight **myopic overcorrection** and follow up closely for aphakic glaucoma and visual development. I will insert an intraocular lens implant calculated for mild residual hyperopia when the patient is between one and two years old.

Note:

- In unilateral cataracts, avoid surgery before six weeks of age (balance between increased risk of aphakic glaucoma versus development of visual impairment). In bilateral cases, operate simultaneously one–two weeks apart and prescribe aphakic glasses postoperatively.
- Intraocular lens should be implanted between one and two years of age (minimum six months of age). Posterior capsulotomy should be performed for patients below seven to eight years of age or patients who are uncooperative, e.g. patients with Down's syndrome.
- Indication of anterior vitrectomy: visual axis opacification due to migration of anterior lens cells to the anterior hyloid.

Q Question 12.4 What are the Difficulties or Complications of a Pediatric Cataract Operation?

Complications can be divided into **intraoperative, early postoperative,** and **late postoperative** complications. Intraoperative risks and difficulties include **risk of general anesthesia, tight space due to small anterior chamber, soft sclera, elastic anterior capsule whereby capsulorrhexis** is difficult to perform with increased risk of **runout,** and **solid anterior hyaloid phase.** Early postoperative complications include **infection, hypotony, raised intraocular pressures, retinal detachments,** and **corneal edema.** Late postoperative complications include **corneal decompensation, glaucoma (especially if left aphakic), posterior capsular opacification, prolonged inflammation, lens decentration, myopic shift, retinal detachment,** and **need for treatment of amblyopia.**

Q Question 12.5 What are the Poor Prognostic Factors?

Poor prognostic factors include **long-standing cataracts, dense cataracts involving central optical zone, presence of strabismus, poor visual acuity,** and **lack of stereopsis.**

Q Question 12.6 What are the Indications for Cataract Surgery?

Indications include **poor fixation, strabismus, poor visual acuity despite refractive correction** and **patching, poor fundal view,** and **dense cataract occupying central 3 mm optical zone.**

Q **Question 13** Viva Stem: 8-day-old Infant referred by the Neonatologist for Bilateral Red Eyes and Discharge. How would you Manage?

In an eight-day-old infant with red eyes, I will **exclude sight-threatening** causes such as **ophthalmia neonatorium** (conjunctivitis in less than one month) secondary to bacterial or viral infections (unlikely chemical as it is already eight days after delivery), **congenital glaucoma, infective keratitis**, and **uveitis** as well as common causes such as **epiblepharon** and **corneal abrasion** (presentation of congenital nasolacrimal duct obstruction is unlikely at this age). I will examine the patient's history for duration of onset, progression, trauma, birth history, any maternal infections, or sexually transmitted disease. I will check for relative afferent pupillary defect and red reflex; check the lids for entropion/ectropion/epiblepharon and presence of purulent discharge; check the anterior segment for infiltrates, follicles, hazy cornea, increased corneal diameter, anterior chamber activity, keratic precipitates, and hypopyon; check the intraocular pressure; and perform a dilated fundal examination for tumors or increased cup-disc ratio.

I will investigate by taking **a swab and sending for microscopy and cultures for chocolate agar, chlamydia immunofluorescence (looking for intracellular inclusion bodies)**, and **polymerase chain reaction**. If there is maternal history of gonococcal infection or if the suspicion is high, I will co-manage the patient with the pediatrician and start the patient on intravenous **ceftriaxone 50 mg/kg/day** in divided doses in the absence of contraindications. I will ensure frequent eye toilet to remove the discharges and start **topical erythromycin eye drops**. I will also start the patient on chlamydia treatment of oral **erythroymycin 50 mg/kg/day** in divided doses (four times a day) for two weeks, refer the parents to the infectious disease specialist for contact tracing and screening, and start the **parents on ceftriaxone 1 g twice a day or IM ceftazidime and oral single dose of azithromycin 1 g**. (If the mother has a sexually transmitted disease and the baby needs prophylaxis, use 2.5% providone iodine one drop followed by topical erythromycin and intramuscular penicillin G. If suspicion of herpes is high, give acyclovir syrup 30 mg/kg/day in three divided doses for two weeks. Common bacterial causes include gonococcal, chlamydia, staph, strep, hemophilus, and enterococcus.)

Note: A child with **photophobia**: congenital causes include glaucoma, aniridia, anterior segment dysgenesis, congenital hereditary endothelial dystrophy, congenital cataracts, albinism, and cone dystrophies (older children). Acquired causes include corneal abrasion, poor ocular surface egepiblepharon, infective keratitis, and uveitis.

> **Q** **Question 14.1** Viva Stem: Parents of a 2-year-old Child are Worried about a Growth over his Left Eye (see Figure 7.13). They would like to seek Treatment for the Lesion. What is your Impression, what will you Examine, and What History will you Take?

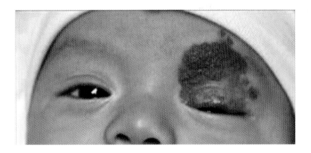

Figure 7.13 Left upper lid capillary hemangioma with resultant mechanical ptosis obscuring the visual axis. This patient is at risk of developing amblyopia if the lesion is left untreated.

This is the partial facial photo of the child. There is a **strawberry nevus** of the left upper lid which is a **capillary hemangioma** causing partial ptosis that appears to be obscuring the visual axis. I will lift up the lids to assess the Hirschberg light reflex. There is no significant **proptosis**. I will check the **visual acuity by age-appropriate method, relative afferent pupillary defect, extraocular movements, intraocular pressure, and anterior segment** for exposure, perform a **dilated fundal examination** for disc swelling or pallor, perform **a cycloplegic refraction** by retinoscopy, and examine systemically for associated features of **high output cardiac failure** (such as **Maffucci syndrome — enchondromas** and **Kasabach-Merritt syndrome — consumptive thrombocytopenia**). I will examine the patient's history for duration of onset, progression, and whether the lesion increases on crying.

> **Q** **Question 14.2** What are Some Complications that Could Arise in the Patient in Question 14.1 and how would you Manage them?

Complications can be divided into **systemic** or **ocular**. Systemic complications include high output cardiac failure, consumptive thrombocytopenia, and anemia, as well as visceral hemangiomas and enchondromas. **Ocular** complications include **astigmatism with meri-donial amblyopia** and **occlusion amblyopia** as the lesion involves the visual axis, as well as **proptosis, exposure,** and **compressive optic neuropathy**. Management can be divided into systemic and ocular. Systemically, I will co-manage the systemic associations in the patient with the pediatrician. Ocular-wise, management can be divided into systemic, which is first-line, and local, treatment. This child will need early treatment to prevent amblyopia. I will get the pediatrician to start the patient on **oral beta-blockers** such as propranolol or **oral steroids** in the absence of contraindications. If these fail, local treatment such as **intralesional steroid injection, radiotherapy, angiographic embolization, or surgery** can be considered.

Note: If there are no complications, most patients can be treated conservatively and monitored. The majority will regress spontaneously by the ages of seven–eight (40% in four years, 70% in seven years).

CHAPTER 8

REFRACTIVE

Q **Question 1.1 OSCE Stem: Examine the Anterior Segment of the Eye as shown in Figure 8.1.**

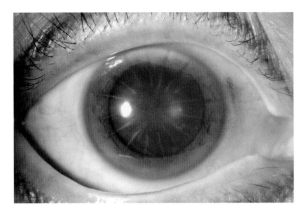

Figure 8.1 16-incision radial keratotomy in a myopic eye.

On examination of the anterior segment of the right eye, the most notable findings are **16 radial keratotomy scars** extending from the periphery toward, but not involving, the visual axis. On casting a slit, the scars are **near full thickness in depth**. The cornea is otherwise clear without evidence of **ectasia, iron line, or anterior stromal haze** (that might suggest photorefractive keratectomy enhancement). The anterior chamber is deep and quiet with a mild nuclear sclerotic lens. On looking down, the patient does not have a trabeculectomy nor glaucoma drainage device implant. Examination of the fellow eye reveals similar findings. I will check the visual acuity and **refractive status**, and perform a dilated fundal examination for **myopic changes, retinal tears**, or **detachments**.

Issues can be divided into **biometry** and **surgical difficulties**. In patients with previous refractive surgery, obtaining accurate biometry and lens calculations could be difficult, and postoperative **refractive surprise** and **hyperopic shift** can occur. Correction of radial keratotomy-induced astigmatism could be challenging as well. I will use newer-generation biometry formulas such as Haigis-L or ASCRS calculator to calculate the required lens power, aiming for a more myopic endpoint of –1 diopter. Intraoperatively, the cataract incision has to **avoid the radial cuts** to avoid gape, rupture, fish mouthing with subsequent poor healing, and high induced astigmatism. I will perform the cataract surgery under regional anesthesia with a sclera tunnel. If the wound incision ruptures, I will need to suture the wound immediately.

Note: Biometric options for patients with previous refractive surgeries: Haigis-L formula, Barrett true-K formula, ASCRS website formula, contact lens method, historical method.

Q **Question 2.1 Viva Stem: A 25-year-old would like to be Spectacle-free. Her Refractive Status is OD –4.00/–0.50 x 60 and OS –4.25/–0.25 x 70. What are the Available Options Suitable for her?**

In this young patient with **moderate myopia** and **minimal astigmatism**, options can be divided into **conservative** and **surgical**. Conservative option includes soft and rigid gas permeable **contact lenses**, but they carry an increased risk of infection. Surgical options can be divided into **keratorefractive** and **intraocular surgeries**. Keratorefractive surgeries can be further divided into (1) **advanced surface ablations** such as photorefractive keratectomy (rarely performed nowadays), epi-LASIK, and LASEK; (2) **flap-based** such as LASIK; and (3) **lenticular extraction** such as ReLEX and SMILE. Intraocular surgery includes implantation of **intra-collamer lens** (sulcus-supported).

> Avoid surface ablation in patients > 6 diopter due to increased risk of haze or corneal thickness < 460 μm.
> Avoid LASIK and lenticular extractions in patients > 10 diopter or corneal thickness < 480 μm.

Q **Question 2.2 What are the Advantages of Flap Surgery versus Surface Ablation?**

Patients undergoing flap surgery (i.e. LASIK) have faster visual recovery, less postoperative discomfort, less stromal haze, shorter duration of postoperative medications and lower risk of infection. Patients undergoing surface ablation have less dry eyes, lower risk of postoperative ectasia, and do not have flap-related complications such as decentration, striae, interface haze, dislodgement, and diffuse lamellar keratitis.

Q **Question 2.3** **Who would be more Suitable for Advanced Surface Ablation?**

Patients who have more significant dry eyes, thinner corneas or residual stromal bed (i.e. greater degree of ablation required), basement membrane dystrophy, or anterior stromal scars.

Q **Question 2.4** **What are the Contraindications of LASIK?**

The contraindications can be divided into **patient** and **ocular** factors. Patient factors include young patients (where the refractive status has not stabilized yet, preferably > 21 years of age), pregnant or breastfeeding patients, history of collagen vascular disease, and poorly controlled diabetics. Ocular factors include patient with keratoconus or forme fruste keratoconus, severe dry eyes, thin corneas or thin residual stromal beds, history of glaucoma, and previous herpetic corneal infections.

Q **Question 3.1** **Viva Stem: A 22-year-old Patient would like to be Spectacle-free. His Refractive Status is OD –15.00/–0.50 x 90 and OS –15.00/–0.25 x 80. What are his Options?**

In this young patient with pathological myopia more than 10 diopter in each eye, he would be a **high risk candidate** for flap-based keratorefractive surgery unless he has pre-existing thick corneas. Likewise, he will **not be suitable for lenticular extraction** or **advanced surface ablation procedures**. Options for him can be divided into (1) **conservative** — mainly, the use of **contact lenses** and (2) **surgical** — implantation of **intra-collamer lens**.

Q **Question 3.2** **If All Examinations are Normal, What Investigations would you perform for the Patient in Question 3.1?**

As this patient will require implantation of an intra-collamer lens, I will check the **manifest** and **cycloplegic refraction, anterior chamber depth**, and **white-to-white distance**.

Q Question 3.3 How would you Counsel a Patient for Intra-Collamer Lens Implantation?

I will advise him as follows:

"Sir, you will be undergoing an operation where we will be creating a small wound in the cornea. Through this wound we will be inserting an intraocular lens, placing it in front of your own natural lens. This may have to be done under general anesthesia to avoid sudden movements. It is a generally safe operation but there are some risks associated with it. The general risks include risk of anesthesia, excessive bleeding, infection, and blindness. Specific risks related to this operation include sudden rise in intraocular pressure after the operation, glaucoma, prolonged inflammation (uveitis-glaucoma-hyphema syndrome), and refractive surprise that might require exchange of the lens, as well as development of cataract in the future. You will need to be on long-term follow-up after the operation."

Q Question 4.1 Viva Stem: A Patient recently underwent LASIK Surgery. He was noted to have the following findings 2 months after the Operation (see Figure 8.2). The Patient is Otherwise Asymptomatic, with a Best-Corrected Visual Acuity of 6/4.5 OU. How would you Manage such a Patient?

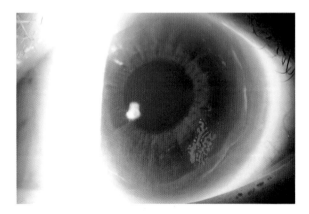

Figure 8.2 Left epithelial ingrowth after LASIK surgery that does not involve the visual axis.

This is the sclerotic scatter anterior segment photograph of the patient's left eye showing the presence of a LASIK flap with a well-defined patch of **grayish geographic opacity** suggestive of a **nest of epithelial ingrowth** at the 5 o'clock mid-peripheral region not involving the visual axis, located about 2 mm from the flap edge. I will cast a slit to determine its depth, look for **rolled corneal flap margins**, and stain with **fluorescein looking for staining** (areas of epithelial fistula) **or pooling** (areas of elevated or retracted flap). Otherwise the cornea is clear with no evidence of **melt** or **haze**. I will examine the contralateral eye, check the visual acuity and refractive status, and examine the fundus for myopic changes.

Note: Haze develops peripheral to the flap edge as flap pulls away in severe epithelial ingrowth, leaving the exposed stromal bed in contact with the overlying epithelium.

Q | Question 4.2 How would you Manage the Patient in Question 4.1?

Management depends on the **severity** and **location** of the epithelial ingrowth. In this patient, as the extent is small, localized and away from the visual axis with good visual acuity, I will monitor the patient closely at **weekly intervals for a month** with **serial corneal topography** and **photograph** and continue **topical steroid therapy**, watching for progression. If there is no further progression, I will resume routine follow-up. If it progresses and involves the visual axis or it is associated with complications such as **flap necrosis** and **significant irregular astigmatism**, the patient will need a **flap re-lift and debridement with suturing of the flap** (to reduce recurrence). I will place a **bandage contact lens**, start topical antibiotics and steroids in the absence of contraindications, and monitor closely for recurrence.

Note: Treat based on Probst/Machat grading criteria.

Q | Question 5.1 Viva Stem: A Young 25-year-old Patient underwent LASIK three months ago and now Complains of Gradually Progressive Painless Worsening of his Vision in the Left Eye over the past two months. What are the Possible Causes?

Possible differentials can be divided into sight-threatening and non-sight-threatening causes. Sight-threatening causes include ectasia (most important), steroid-induced glaucoma, pressure-induced stromal keratitis, and epithelial ingrowth with corneal flap melt. Non-sight-threatening causes include most commonly dry eyes, regression, and corneal flap haze.

> Provide differentials that are progressive and painless occurring at about two to three months postoperatively, i.e. differentials such as under/over correction, diffuse lamellar keratitis, infective keratitis, or decentered ablation are not applicable.

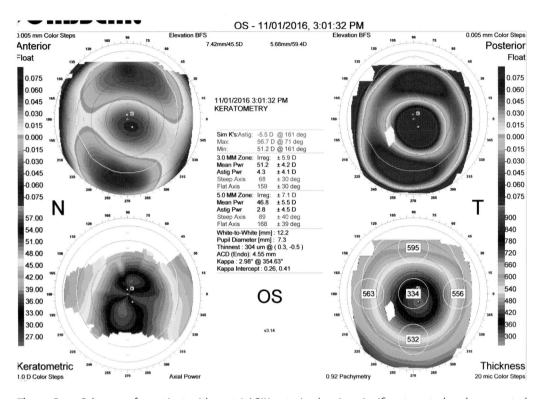

Figure 8.3 Orb scan of a patient with post-LASIK ectasia showing significant central and paracentral thinning with increased irregular astigmatism.

This is the orb scan of the patient's left eye. There is **elevation of both the anterior** and **posterior float centrally above the best fit sphere**. On the keratometric map, there is a **skewed bow-tie appearance with inferior steepening**. There is **corresponding inferior paracentral thinning** on the pachymetric map as well. The **Sim K** is increased at −5.5 diopter at 161 degrees. Both the 3.0-mm zone and 5.0-mm zone have increased astigmatism and the **thinnest area measures 304 μm**. In view of the history of previous LASIK surgery, he has left **post-LASIK ectasia**.

Q **Question 5.3 How would you Manage the Patient in Question 5.2?**

I will examine the patient's history for previous ocular diseases, connective tissue disease, and family history of keratoconus. I will examine the left eye for **significant stromal**

scarring, examine the **contralateral eye for features of keratoconus**, and perform an orb scan for the right eye. Management of post-LASIK ectasia can be divided into **conservative** and **surgical**. In this patient, I will try conservative measures such as refractive correction with **glasses** or contact lenses such as **rigid gas permeable lenses** (he is unlikely to tolerate toric soft contact lens due to the high astigmatism) and monitor the patient closely. Indications for optical keratoplasty for this patient include **intolerance to contact lenses, signs of progression or poor vision secondary to significant stromal scarring,** or **severe astigmatism**. Options of optical keratoplasty include full thickness penetrating keratoplasty and lamellar keratoplasty. (Collagen crosslinking is contraindicated in this patient due to severe thinning with corneal thickness < 400 μm.)

Q **Question 6.1** Viva Stem: A 50-year-old Patient with Bilateral Mild Cataracts has a Best-Corrected Visual Acuity of 6/9 ou and Refractive Error of OD −3.00/−1.00 x 90, OS −2.00/−0.50 x 90. Examination shows her Condition is Otherwise Unremarkable. She would like to explore her Options with regard to Refractive Correction. How would you Manage such a Patient?

In this patient with mild cataracts, good visual acuity, and low myopia, her options can be divided into conservative and surgical. Conservative options include glasses (progressive, bifocal, or reading glasses) and contact lenses. Surgical options include bilateral LASIK aiming for emmetropia with reading glasses and monovision LASIK. She is not an ideal candidate for inlays which is best reserved for **non-dominant eyes with emmetropia or low hyperopia**. She is also not suitable for cataract surgery as she has mild cataracts with good best-corrected visual acuity. I will explain to the patient that she needs to read under strong lighting conditions and that her presbyopia is likely to worsen: she still might require spectacles eventually. I will also ask her to consider a cataract operation with the appropriate intraocular lens implantation when the cataract is visually significant.

Note: Multifocal/presbyopic LASIK is rarely performed in our center as it is only a one-off correction with effects of increased haloes and glare.

Q **Question 6.2** What are the Issues with Monovision?

Monovision is not suitable for everyone. Disadvantages of monovision include reduction in stereopsis, difficulty tolerating anisometropia, need for spectacles for clear vision with both eyes, poorer night vision. It is also not suitable for patients who drive at night, read for prolonged periods of time (results in significant asthenopia), require vision for fine work and sports.

Q **Question 6.3** How would you Manage a Patient who returns several years later with Bilateral Visually Significant Cataracts? (She has been using reading glasses in the meantime.)

As the patient has bilateral visually significant cataracts, she will benefit from bilateral sequential cataract surgery with intraocular lens implant. Choice of intraocular lens correction includes bilateral monofocal lenses aiming for emmetropia with or without toric correction (mainly for the right eye), monovision, bilateral multifocal intraocular lenses with or without toric correction as well as extended depth of focus lenses. I will explain in detail the risks and benefits of each option and emphasize that she might still require spectacle correction eventually for both distance and near vision.

Issues Associated with Multifocal Intraocular Lens

- Reduced night vision and contrast
- Glare and halos
- Quality of vision is poorer compared to monofocal lens
- Requires good lighting
- Poorer intermediate vision (unless trifocal lens was implanted)
- Should be implanted bilaterally
- Spectacles might still be required for distance and near vision
- Intolerance might necessitate intraocular lens exchange
- Multifocal intraocular lens should be avoided if there are intra-operative complications e.g. posterior capsular rupture

CHAPTER 9

MISCELLANEOUS

Q Question 1 Viva Stem: How would you work up a Patient prior to Initiation of Intravenous Steroid Therapy and how would you Monitor the Patient?

I will first **admit** the patient. Investigation can be divided into blood tests, urine tests, and other miscellaneous tests. For blood tests, I will order a full blood count for raised white blood cells, erythrocyte sedimentation rate, C-reactive protein, renal panel and liver panel, and capillary blood glucose. An **Infective screen** will include human immunodeficiency virus, hepatitis B and C, syphilis VDRL and LIA-IgG IgM. Urine tests include urine culture and urine full examination microscopy elements. Miscellaneous tests include chest X-ray (especially for tuberculosis), mantoux test, electrocardiogram, and blood pressure assessment.

I will put the patient on **continuous monitoring of vitals** and **electrocardiogram during the infusion,** checking the **serum potassium four hours after the infusion,** and monitoring the vitals (temperature and blood pressure) four times a day, capillary blood glucose three times a day, and at 10 p.m., examine the stool chart.

Q Question 2.1 Viva Stem: A Construction Worker was Drilling when he felt a Sudden Sharp Pain

This is the photograph of the patient's right eye. There is a **full-thickness laceration** at 5 o'clock extending from the cornea to the sclera associated with a prolapsed iris, corectopia, and shallow anterior chamber. The rest of the cornea is clear and the conjunctiva is injected with surrounding subconjunctival hemorrhage. There are neither obvious lid nor punctal injuries seen. The lens appears intact with absence of focal cataract. There is no obvious foreign body seen in the photo.

Penetrating globe injury is an ocular emergency. Principles of management of globe trauma are to exclude life-threatening and sight-threatening injuries, restore normal globe anatomy, remove intraocular foreign bodies, treat any underlying infection, treat long-term complications, and undertake visual rehabilitation. I will examine the

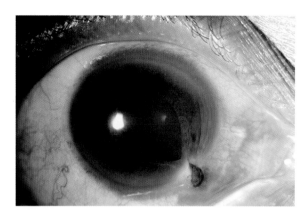
Figure 9.1   Right corneoscleral full-thickness laceration with iris prolapse.

patient's history of onset of injury, mechanism, whether the patient had any protective gear, any foreign body removal on route to hospital, and time of last meal and drink. I will also check the patient's past medical history and drug allergies. I will check his **visual acuity** and **relative afferent pupillary defect by the reverse method**. I will check externally for **proptosis** suggestive of retrobulbar hemorrhage and **extraocular movements, crepitus, step deformity,** or **infraorbital hypoesthesia** suggestive of orbital wall fracture in blunt trauma cases. I will examine the anterior segment **gently,** checking closely for intraocular foreign bodies, iridodialysis, and focal cataracts (which suggests a breach of the anterior capsule) that is otherwise not obvious on the photograph, examine the fundus if possible for vitreous hemorrhage intraocular foreign bodies, retinal tear, and detachment (look for retinal dialysis and optic nerve swelling as well in blunt trauma cases).

I will inform patient of **guarded prognosis** and investigate by checking **preoperative tests** such as full blood count and renal panel. I will order a chest X-ray as well as an electrocardiogram. **I will shield the eye, inject intramuscular tetanus, start intravenous ciprofloxacin 400 mg twice a day in the absence of contraindications, keep the patient nil by mouth, and perform a computer tomography scan of the orbits with fine cuts to localize any foreign body and to exclude orbital fractures** (do not perform magnetic resonance imaging as there might be presence of metallic foreign bodies).

I will inform the anesthetist to perform the surgery under **general anesthesia, avoiding depolarizing agents**. Perioperatively, I will swab the wound and send for cultures and microscopy. Intraoperatively, I will clean and drape with **chlorhexidine** to the skin, retract the lids with Jeffrey's lid retractor or lid traction sutures, and perform an exploratory conjunctival peritomy. If the wound extends under the rectus muscle, I will need to disinsert the rectus muscle to determine the extent of the wound. I will then reform the anterior chamber using viscoelastic through an anterior chamber paracentesis wound, reposit viable tissues and excise non-viable tissues (absence of bleeding), check for vitreous and perform sponge vitrectomy, appose the limbus first with **10/0 nylon,** then close the **cornea** using **10/o nylon** aiming for **90% depth water-tight sutures** that are **longer, more widely spaced at the periphery, and shorter closer apart toward the centre**. I will then close the sclera with 8/o nylon. **I will assess for leakage using fluorescein and augment with sutures or corneal glue (cyanoacrylic) if required**.

I will then close the conjunctiva with **8/o vicryl** and inject cefazolin gentamicin; place a **bandage contact lens** and start the patient on intensive topical fortified broad-spectrum antibiotics; admit the patient for close monitoring for complications such as **infection, wound leakage, hypotony, and sympathetic ophthalmia of the contralateral eye**; and put on an eye shield. I will track the cultures urgently over the next few days and consider steroids once the cultures are known.

Q Question 2.2 How do you perform Disinsertion of the Rectus in the event of Globe Trauma?

Disinsertion of the rectus muscle is required when lacerations extend under the rectus muscle. I will **disinsert the rectus muscle to assess the posterior extent of the globe laceration**. After performing generous conjunctival peritomy, I will first hook the rectus muscle with a squint hook and spread it over a Chavasse hook, then use a double-armed **6/o vicryl**, tag the muscle 1 mm from the insertion site with **interlocking sutures, splitting muscle into thirds**. I will clamp the two suture ends using a bulldog clamp. I will disinsert the muscle using a straight Strabismus scissors between the tag and the insertion site, explore the wound as posteriorly as possible, and suture the scleral laceration with **8/o nylon** as posteriorly as possible. I will reinsert the rectus muscle to the stump using 6/o vicryl.

Q Question 2.3 What type of Lacerations could you Observe and not Repair?

I will observe lacerations that are partial thickness without wound gape as well as small self-sealing, shelving full-thickness lacerations that have re-epithelized with absence of intraocular foreign bodies and with Seidel negative results (usually five to seven days old). In patients with severe trauma and extensive tissue loss with no possibility of vision, I will consider the patient for primary enucleation in consultation with two senior doctors.

Q Question 2.4 How would you Classify Globe Trauma?

Globe injuries can be classified based on the **Birmingham Eye Trauma Terminology (BETT) system**. Injuries are divided into closed and open globe injuries. Closed globe injuries can be further subdivided into contusion and lamellar lacerations. Open globe injuries can be further subdivided into rupture (blunt trauma) and lacerations which include penetrating, perforating, and intraocular foreign bodies.

Options of closure include bridging mattress sutures or purse string sutures.

Q **Question 3.1** OSCE Stem: Please Examine this Patient's eyes. (see Figures 9.2A and 9.2B)

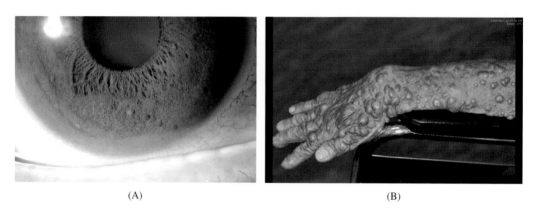

(A)   (B)

Figure 9.2 (A) Lisch nodule. (B) Multiple neurofibromas. This patient has neurofibromatosis type I. In a darkened examination room, candidates might rush into examining the eye and miss the gross systemic lesions as shown in photo B. It is always prudent to take a quick look at the patient before focusing on the eye.

On examination of the anterior segment of the patient's right eye, there are multiple nodules of varying sizes on the iris distributed in the mid-peripheries that are non-pigmented. These are likely to be **Lisch nodules**. Differentials include **Busacca nodules** but there is **absence of posterior synechiae, peripheral anterior synechiae, or keratic precipitates, and the anterior chamber is quiet**. There are associated **prominent corneal nerves** but no **ectropion uvea**. Otherwise the cornea is clear, the anterior chamber is deep, and the patient is phakic. There are no iris transillumination defects, and no **trabeculectomy** or **glaucoma drainage device**. Examination of the fellow eye reveals similar findings. This patient has bilateral Lisch nodules likely associated with **neurofibromatosis type 1**.

I will assess the optic nerve function by checking the visual acuity, relative afferent pupillary defect, color vision, and confrontational visual fields; check the intraocular pressure and extraocular movements; check for pulsatile proptosis with the Hertel's exophthalmometer secondary to sphenoid wing dysplasia, perform a dilated fundal examination for optic disc pallor, cupping, or **optociliary shunts** as well as **choroidal naevus, melanoma, or astrocytomas**. On examination of the upper limbs, there are multiple neurofibromas. I will examine systemically for axillary freckling, plexiform fibromas, café au lait spots, and pseudoarthrosis, and examine the patient's history for first-degree relative involvement. (Other associated abnormalities include vertebral abnormalities such as scoliosis and hypertension.)

Q Question 3.2 What are some Causes of Café Au Lait Spots?

Causes include neurofibromatosis type 1, type 2, tuberous sclerosis, Duane's syndrome, and McCune-Albright syndrome.

Q Question 3.3 What is a Potentially Life-threatening Condition associated with Neurofibromatosis Type 1?

Neurofibromatosis type 1 is associated with pheochromocytoma which is potentially life-threatening.

Q Question 4 Examination of the Anterior Segment of a Patient below (see Figures 9.3A and 9.3B).

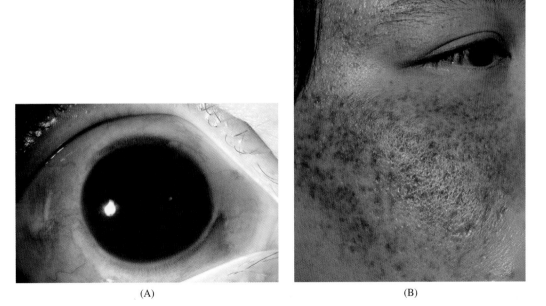

(A)　　　　　　　　　　　　　　　　(B)

Figure 9.3　(A) Slate gray pigmentation in a patient with melanosis. (B) Facial pigmentation in the V1 and V2 dermatome. This patient has oculodermal melanocytosis i.e. nevus of Ota.

On examination of the anterior segment of the patient's right eye, there are large patches of **slate gray subepithelial hyperpigmentation** sparing the nasal region suggestive of **melanosis**. On examination of the anterior segment, there are **mammillations**/harmatomas on the iris with **hyperpigmentation**. Examination of the contralateral eye shows that it is normal indicating the presence of **heterochromia** between the two eyes. On systemic examination, the patient also has **hyperpigmentation of the skin in the V1 and V2 dermatome**. The patient has **nevus of Ota**. I will check the visual acuity and relative afferent pupillary defect, perform a gonioscopy and check the **intraocular pressure**, perform a dilated fundal examination for increased cup-disc ratio and choroidal melanoma, check for proptosis using Hertel's exophthalmometer for **cavernous hemangioma**, and check systemically for **hyperpigmentation of the scapula (nevus of Ito)**.

Q Question 5 OSCE Stem Examine the Anterior Chamber (see Figure 9.4).

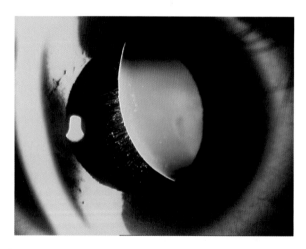

Figure 9.4 Ectopia lentis in a patient with Marfan's syndrome.

On examination of the anterior segment of the left eye, there is **superior temporal subluxation** of the crystalline clear lens with **zonular attachments** seen with **associated phacodonesis**. The anterior chamber is deep and quiet with **no evidence of pupil block** and there is **absence of vitreous** in the anterior chamber. The cornea is clear with no evidence of **keratoconus**. There are no signs of **previous trauma** (e.g. iridodialysis or iris sphincter rupture) or features of **pseudoexfoliation**. There are no transillumination defects on retro-illumination as well (peripheral iridotomy for pupil block).

Examination of the right eye reveals similar findings. The patient has bilateral ectopia lentis. I will check the visual acuity and intraocular pressure, lay the patient supine to assess the degree of posterior displacement, and perform a dilated fundal examination for features of high myopia or retinal tears or detachment. On systemic examination, the patient **is tall and thin with arachnodactylyl**. I will examine for other features of **Marfan's syndrome** such as scoliosis, aortic regurgitation, hyperlaxity of joints, high arched palate, and pectus excavatum. This patient has bilateral ectopia lentis secondary to Marfan's syndrome.

Note: Look for systemic features of homocystinuria and Weill-Marchesani syndrome in the absence of features of Marfan's syndrome. Treatment of homocystinuria: vitamine B6 (pyridoxine), B12, and folate; restrict methionine, anti-platelets or anti-coagulation.

Causes of Bilateral Aphakia		
Surgical	**Non-Surgical**	
Adult	**Primary**	**Secondary**
• Intracapsular cataract extraction	• Ectopic lentis et pupillae	
• Retinal detachment with silicone oil	• Familial ectopic lentis (AD)	*Systemic*
• Clear lens extraction for high myopia	• Idiopathic	• Chromosomal (trisomy)
		• Connective tissue disorders (Ehlers-Danlos, Weill-Marchesani, Stickler, Marfan–superior temporal)
Child		• Metabolic (homocystinuria — interior nasal, hyperlycinemia — interior nasal, sulphite oxidase deficiency — universal)
• Cataract in juvenile idiopathic arthritis		
• Cataract < One year old		*Ocular*
		• Ocular developmental disorders (big eyes and cornea — megalocornea, bulpthalmos, iris anomalies — aniridia (keratoconus), uvelcoloboma, corectopia)
		• Ocular diseases/acquired (trauma, uveitis, PXF, hypermature cataracts, anterior uveal tumors)

INDEX

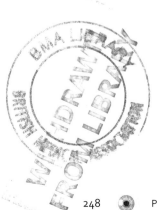

Practical Guide to Viva and OSCE in Ophthalmology Examinations